"David VanDrunen's stimulating book on bioethics is a great help to us as we wrestle through some very difficult issues in our day. Discussing everything from cloning, contraception, and stem cell research to health care for the incapacitated and how to decide if treatment should be pursued, VanDrunen shows himself an able guide and wise mentor. These are difficult issues, but he addresses them in a thoughtful and accessible way. One of the most promising aspects of this book is VanDrunen's consistent engagement in fresh biblical exegesis, while also drawing from a natural law tradition, all the while maintaining a focus that is both churchly and relevant for today."

—**Kelly M. Kapic**, Associate Professor of Theological Studies,
Covenant College

"*Bioethics and the Christian Life* provides a much-needed guide to the difficult area of Christian clinical bioethics. While many well-meaning Christians present bioethics for marionette puppets (with God pulling the strings) and secularists claim that we are the masters of our fate and captains of our soul, VanDrunen does the hard work of guiding his reader to exercise autonomy responsibly within God's revealed will in the Bible. Here is rich guidance to help the patient, family member, pastor, or clinician to think Christianly and find biblically sound answers to the vexing problems of bioethics."

—**Thomas W. Ziegler**, MD, FACP, Clinical Professor of Medicine (retired),
University of California San Diego and VA Medical Center, San Diego,
California; Ruling Elder, New Life Presbyterian Church (PCA),
La Mesa, California

"Dr. VanDrunen adds significantly and positively to the bioethical conversation in ways that will help every pastor and every thoughtful Christian to think through issues of life and death. He interacts with contemporary biotechnology and bioethics and asks the difficult questions, giving thoughtful, nuanced answers based on sound orthodox theology and Christian virtue. What distinguishes this book is that particular issues are not approached in isolation from the biblical goal of a well-lived Christian life. Fixed moral truths of God's law do not always yield clear answers to every ethical question, but biblical wisdom enables the Christian to navigate the difficulties and avoid facile answers. VanDrunen is firm in his conclusions when scripture speaks clearly, but he is wisely wary of being dogmatic where scripture is silent. I highly recommend this book. As a primer in Christian ethics it should be the text for a required Christian education course in every church."

—**Gregory Edward Reynolds**, pastor, Amoskeag Presbyterian Church,
Manchester, New Hampshire; author, *The Word Is Worth a Thousand
Pictures: Preaching in the Electronic Age*; editor, *Ordained Servant:
A Journal for Church Officers*

BIOETHICS
AND THE
CHRISTIAN LIFE

BIOETHICS
AND THE
CHRISTIAN LIFE

A Guide to Making Difficult Decisions

DAVID VANDRUNEN

:: CROSSWAY WHEATON, ILLINOIS

Bioethics and the Christian Life: A Guide to Making Difficult Decisions
Copyright © 2009 by David VanDrunen

Published by Crossway Books
        a publishing ministry of Good News Publishers
        1300 Crescent Street
        Wheaton, Illinois 60187

Interior design and typesetting by Lakeside Design Plus
Cover design by Josh Dennis
First printing 2009
Printed in the United States of America

Unless otherwise indicated, Scripture quotations are from the ESV® Bible (*The Holy Bible, English Standard Version®*), copyright © 2001 by Crossway Bibles, a publishing ministry of Good News Publishers. Used by permission. All rights reserved.

Scripture quotations marked AT are the author's translation.

All emphases in Scripture quotations have been added.

Trade Paperback ISBN: 978-1-4335-0144-9
PDF ISBN: 978-1-4335-1265-0
MobiPocket ISBN: 978-1-4335-1266-7
ePub ISBN: 978-1-4335-2183-6

Library of Congress Cataloging-in-Publication Data
VanDrunen, David, 1971–
   Bioethics and the Christian life : a guide to making difficult decisions / David
VanDrunen.
      p. cm.
   Includes bibliographical references and index.
   ISBN 978-1-4335-0144-9 (tpb)
     1. Medical ethics—Religious aspects—Christianity. 2. Bioethics—Religious aspects—
Christianity. 3. Christian ethics. I. Title.

   R725.56.V36 2009
   174.2—dc22   2009003977

VP		20	19	18	17	16	15	14	13	12	11	10	09
14	13	12	11	10	9	8	7	6	5	4	3	2	1

CONTENTS

PREFACE

The origins of this book date back several years, to a period when I received an unusual number of requests in a short period of time from churches wishing me to teach on bioethical issues. Though I had done some study and a little teaching and writing on the subject before that time, I never intended to devote a concentrated period of research to or to write a book about bioethics. But the experience of teaching those church seminars and Sunday school classes revealed how many serious questions thoughtful Christians have about life and death issues in general and about the moral questions surrounding new technologies in particular. Those Christians prompted me to do more study on these problems and eventually convinced me—unknowingly to them—that a book like this one might be helpful. I am grateful for Allan Fisher's initial enthusiasm for this project and for the fine experience that I have had working with him and his colleagues at Crossway in bringing this book to publication.

I wish to express my thanks to a number of others as well. First and foremost, to Katherine and Jack for so many things, and especially their ongoing appreciation of and support for the scholarly life. I am also very grateful to the board, faculty, students, and staff at Westminster Seminary California for continuing to provide such a congenial environment for exploring the kinds of theological and pastoral issues that are discussed here. Thanks to those who were willing to read parts or the whole of the manuscript while it was still very much a draft: Matt Tuininga, John Fesko, Tom Ziegler, Lana Korniyenko, Kelly Kapic, Jack Davis, and Calvin Van Reken (and his anonymous assistant). Not long after I drafted the chapters on death and dying that comprise Part 3 of this book, my grandmother, Grace VanDrunen, died on her ninety-fourth birthday. Those who knew her are grateful for her life and I am thankful that my son, her great-grandchild, participated in the final (very brief) conversation that she had on this earth and thereby witnessed a wonderful example of a Christian who died well.

Readers will note that I have written the text without footnotes. A bibliographic essay in the Conclusion provides information about works that I refer to in the text and it lists some other literature that I think is especially noteworthy. Readers are encouraged to see this essay in the Conclusion if they wish to follow up on any sources or to pursue further study of issues considered within.

Introduction

THE CHRISTIAN CONFRONTS BIOETHICS

Human beings have been pondering ethical questions about life and death from a religious perspective for a very long time. Millennia before the advent of fertility drugs God's Old Testament people wrestled with barrenness and sought various solutions, from prayer to concubines. Christians in the early church confronted and rejected the common Greco-Roman practice of abortion, infanticide, and suicide. Medieval- and Reformation-era Christians had no access to modern life-sustaining technology yet wrote numerous treatises on how to die well.

The kinds of questions evoked by the new academic discipline of "bioethics" are therefore perennial. Yet the harvest of new medical technology in the past generation has brought issues of life and death to a level of difficulty, importance, and promise never before seen in human history. The new technology holds great promise because it offers possibilities for treating ailments and prolonging life in previously unimaginable ways. Great enemies of human flourishing—disease and death—remain undefeated, but they seem increasingly manageable. There has never been a better time to get sick than the present. But with the benefits of human ingenuity come the eerie forebodings of a future that is less humane, not more. The same powers that provide remedies for infertility enable researchers to create embryos as a disposable source of pluripotent stem cells. The ability to manipulate the human genetic code can be harnessed not only for keeping inheritable diseases from the next generation but also for producing designer babies destined to be taller, faster, and smarter than their classmates. Techniques for treating life-threatening illnesses that can restore people to health can also preserve people in vegetative states for decades at great emotional and financial cost to family and society. Many proponents of the new technology denounce those who would stifle research and rob society of its benefits because of quaint moral scruples. Others issue dire warnings about a frightening brave new world that will emerge if scientific technology is not constrained by ethical boundaries. Battles are waged on ballots and in courts about what activities to ban and which research to fund. Families are divided about whether to pursue in vitro fertilization and whether to pull the plug on grandma.

Where do Christians stand in relation to such volatile matters? What difference does Christian commitment make to one's perspective on these issues of life and death? For many Christians of a traditional, conservative bent such bioethical controversies rouse strong feelings and inspire social activism. Like the early Christians we sense our entrenchment in a so-called culture of death and seek to renew respect for all human life, even in its earliest and latest stages. Against the subtle and overt forms of moral relativism that chip away at the foundations of humane civilization we proclaim to the world that many activities are simply wrong.

But the relation of Christian conviction—even of traditional and conservative variety—to contemporary bioethics is in fact much more complicated than suggested in the previous paragraph. Many Christians firmly committed to moral absolutes and troubled by attempts to blur distinctions between right and wrong have found themselves genuinely puzzled by ethical choices that medical technology has thrust in their path. However clear certain matters of abortion or assisted suicide may seem to them, they have found decisions about remedying infertility or discontinuing treatment for a dying relative to be ethically confusing. Under the surface of several high-profile and seemingly easy bioethical issues are a host of matters that appeal to cherished values in conflicting directions and therefore offer no immediately obvious moral answers.

Most Christian couples, for example, have no qualms in principle about seeking medical help when they are unable to conceive children over an extended period of time. These same couples, however, usually also have a sense—even if they struggle to articulate exactly why—that there are boundaries beyond which the quest to have a child should not go. But what precisely are the moral issues at stake, what are these boundaries, and what are the ethical consequences of transgressing them? Most Christians concur that assisting a suicide is morally evil, but they also shrink from the conclusion that they are obligated to do absolutely everything to preserve their own or others' lives as long as possible. But where does one cross the line between allowing death to take its natural and inevitable course and becoming complicit in someone's death due to failure to fight for life? Scripture provides no explicit instruction for making such determinations, and oftentimes trusted pastors and counselors offer conflicting advice. In such situations moral action is doubly difficult: Christians need not only the courage to do what they know is right but also the insight and wisdom to figure out what is right in the first place.

The Purpose of This Book: Bioethics in the Midst of the Christian Life

The present book is written to address these problems. It explores how ordinary Christians, in the midst of the lives that they are called to live in Christ, may come to a better understanding of how to respond to the bioethical questions that confront them, their families, and their fellow believers in the church. This book is not a diatribe against contemporary woes such as the culture of death or the dehumanization of medicine (however much of a concern these things are). Neither is it a rousing call to social and political action on the part of Christians concerned about troubling cultural trends (however beneficial such action might be). I will be grateful if this book proves helpful for understanding contemporary bioethics culture wars and useful for those involved in public debates about bioethics, but these are not its chief concern. Instead I hope first and foremost to offer encouragement and guidance for Christians who seek, in the face of the morally confusing options presented by modern medical technology, to grow in the knowledge of Christian truth and in their practice of the Christian life in ways that prepare them to make personal bioethical decisions with godliness and wisdom.

In light of this I hope to address several overlapping audiences. This book is for all sorts of thoughtful, ordinary Christians who seek to be faithful as they confront issues of life and death in their individual and family lives. It is also intended to help pastors, elders, and counselors who will be increasingly solicited for help in making bioethical decisions. I have also written to facilitate moral reflection among physicians, nurses, and other Christians who work in the health-care system, for whom some of these issues are professional as well as personal. Finally, I hope that this book will be useful to students who are being introduced to the discipline of bioethics.

In treating bioethical issues within the context of the broader Christian life, I am trying to avoid the tendency to confront these issues as discrete moral problems. In other words, I am resisting the temptation to deal with bioethical issues as stand-alone dilemmas isolated from the many moral choices that precede and follow them. Questions are often posed in the abstract: Should a woman pregnant with quadruplets selectively abort two fetuses in order to give the other two a better chance of survival? May an unmarried woman eager to have children let herself be artificially inseminated with the sperm of an anonymous donor? Must a caregiver administer antibiotics to fight an infection in his comatose father when his father is already dying from cancer? Such questions, I argue, should not be considered in the abstract, apart from a person's broader moral life.

This is true, first, because our lives are a connected whole, and the decisions that we make in one situation often determine the kinds of choices that we will face later and affect the way that we resolve those choices. This book certainly does not promise that a little proactive conduct will prevent the necessity of making difficult bioethical decisions. But on some occasions particular bioethical dilemmas are a direct result of previous choices that were either overtly sinful or at least risky and foolish. On other occasions making the wrong decision in the midst of a bioethical crisis leads to another, and even more difficult, crisis later. What sorts of decisions in response to infertility, for example, may have created the moral and emotional hardship of having four struggling fetuses *in utero* or of having to decide what to do with ten frozen embryos whose mother has suddenly died? Proverbs 22:3 counsels us to take cover when we see danger approaching. Wise action now may prevent a bioethical crisis later.

Second, and closely related to the previous matter, is the importance of virtue. One of the chief reasons why we ought to examine individual moral decisions in the light of our broader moral lives is because each one of us has a certain character. People facing difficult bioethical dilemmas face them not as blank slates but as people with certain virtues and vices, that is, with various character traits that orient them toward good or evil. Today ethics is often reduced to a concern about external actions. Through most of Western history, however, ethicists believed that questions of virtue are just as important as rules of conduct, and this is also the biblical perspective. People tend to act according to character. Two individuals may agree in theory that running into a burning building to save a child is the morally proper action, but if one is a man of courage and the other is a coward then most likely only the former will carry out the deed. To put it simply, those who wish to conduct themselves in an externally excellent way must strive to become internally excellent people.

The ramifications for bioethics are profound. Consider a woman diagnosed with an advanced stage of cancer and wrestling with whether to pursue a long-shot, experimental, and burdensome treatment or to let the disease take her life and to die peacefully at home. She confronts that question as a particular kind of person, whose character has been formed through a lifetime of moral experience. Is she a person of contentment? Of courage? Of hope? How does the presence or absence of these virtues bear upon her decision, determining both how she evaluates the attractions of each option and whether she will actually do what she determines is right? Perpetual discontentment, habitual cowardice, and constant despair tend to distort a person's response to a frightening diagnosis and to impede the ability to make a clearheaded and godly decision about treatment.

Hence the present book explores not only what is the right thing to do when confronted with such a difficult bioethical decision, but also what sorts of virtues we should cultivate in order to be prepared to make such choices well. Becoming a morally responsible bioethics decision-maker is the task of a lifetime and cannot be reduced to figuring out the right answer at a particular moment of crisis. Bioethical decisions must be made within the context of lifelong growth in Christian maturity.

Third, this book examines bioethics in light of the broader Christian life rather than as a series of discrete moral problems because many bioethical decisions simply do not have one absolutely binding right or wrong answer. Such decisions depend upon the wisdom and judgment of a particular person acting within a unique set of life circumstances. A good example is the scenario presented above concerning the woman facing experimental and burdensome cancer treatment. The immediate reaction of some readers may have been strongly in favor of pursuing the treatment: the small chance of recovery overrides the burden of the procedure. Conversely, other readers may have felt instinctively attracted to the choice of forgoing treatment and dying peacefully at home: prolonging life at every cost is not the highest good. Two Christians with similar theological convictions may find themselves inclined in opposite directions and be compelled to admit that there is no simple correct answer that one of them could impose upon the other's conscience.

How should a person make a responsible decision under such circumstances? Even when no universally applicable correct answer exists, many factors may make a particular decision *better* or *worse* in particular circumstances. One choice may be more beneficial for the patient's family, church, or spiritual well-being. One choice may better allow the patient to live—or to finish living—in a way that is consistent with the life that she has lived thus far in her study, work, play, and worship. Thus, faced with the choice whether to receive experimental cancer treatment, she may need to ponder at what stage of life she finds herself: does she have meaningful projects left to accomplish, young children needing her care, or significant responsibilities at church or work? She may also need to consider whether her inclination to pursue one choice over the other is an inclination of courage or of cowardice, of hope or of despair, of love or of selfishness. These and other factors, taken together and reflected upon with wisdom, will contribute to making a morally sound and responsible decision.

Thus far I have tried to elucidate one distinctive aspect of this book: considering bioethical issues in the context of the broader Christian life. One other distinctive aspect of this book deserves mention. As I seek to articulate the nature of Christian faith and life in the chapters that follow, I do so from a Reformed theological perspective, as summarized in documents such as the Westminster Confession of Faith and the Heidelberg Catechism. This should not deter readers with different theological convictions. Most of the doctrines and virtues that play an important role in the forthcoming discussions—such as the image of God, divine sovereignty, resurrection, and faith, hope, and love—will be familiar to Christians from many traditions. Throughout the book, furthermore, I seek to show how all of the doctrines and virtues are grounded in Scripture. In light of this, I aim to reach a wide audience and to be helpful to people from various backgrounds. Nevertheless, one conviction that drives this book is that having a firm and knowledgeable theological foundation is crucial for living the Christian life well, and hence for making bioethical decisions responsibly. This book aims to explain that theological foundation as it emerges from Scripture; and that foundation reflects my Reformed convictions.

The Structure of This Book

The following chapters seek to present many clear and forthright answers, from a biblical Christian perspective, to a number of controversial bioethics questions. Perhaps more importantly, however, they offer Christians a *way of thinking* and a *way of approaching* these questions. No book can anticipate every single bioethical problem that a person will face and thus be a comprehensive handbook of bioethical answers. Much more useful, I believe, is a book that trains Christians how to think better about the moral life and how to become people of better Christian character and virtue—so that they will be better prepared to make their own decisions in a messy and complicated world.

Part 1 lays the theological and ethical foundation for thinking well about bioethics and the Christian life. Chapter 1 addresses the general perspective that Christians should take toward the health-care practice and bioethical debates of the broader world. Christians have a sense that their religious commitments should cause them to think distinctively about bioethics, but what are the ramifications? Should Christians participate in the mainstream health-care system or establish their own Christian medical institutions? Should they participate in public debates about bioethics with non-Christians and, if so, how can they do this faithfully and effectively? Chapters 2 and 3 reflect the fact that Christians will not be prepared to make morally responsible bioethical decisions in their personal lives if they are ignorant of relevant theological truths and fail to pursue the requisite Christian virtues. Chapter 2 discusses a number of Christian doctrines that are particularly pertinent to bioethics. Among these doctrines are divine providence, human nature, suffering, death, and resurrection. Chapter 3 then considers many virtues that should mark the Christian life: faith, hope, love, courage, contentment, and wisdom.

Part 2 concerns issues pertaining to the *beginning of life*, one of the major general areas of bioethics controversy. Chapter 4 focuses upon matters of marriage and procreation. What is the place and importance of marriage for the Christian life? Is being unmarried a good thing, or is it simply a prelude to marriage? How should Christians understand the good of bearing children? May Christians seek *not* to have children and, if so, which means of doing so are morally acceptable? Chapter 5 then turns to the question of assisted reproduction. What sort of attitude should Christians take toward infertility, which is such a trial for so many people? Should Christians pursue fertility treatments and, if so, which ones are morally acceptable? What should Christians think of standard procedures like in vitro fertilization and exotic dreams like cloning? Chapter 6 concludes Part 2 with a lengthy discussion of the value of unborn human life. When does life begin and to what sort of protection are unborn human beings entitled? What should Christians' attitudes be toward socially divisive issues such as abortion and stem-cell research?

Part 3 turns to bioethical issues at the *end of life*, another general area that has provoked difficult and controversial moral questions. Chapter 7 considers the Christian attitude toward death in general, an attitude that should shape the concrete moral choices that arise as death approaches. What does death mean for the Christian in light of the death and resurrection of Christ? How should Christians look at their entire lives as a preparation for death? What concrete steps should Christians take so that death does not take them unawares? Should Christians agree to become organ donors? In chapter 8 I explore whether Christians may ever actively seek their own death or the death of others. How should Christians view suicide? Is the distinction between *killing* and *letting die* a helpful and valid ethical idea? Is there a place for Christians to support euthanasia, that is, the practice of assisted suicide? Finally, chapter 9 considers the very trying questions of accepting and forgoing medical treatment as death approaches. After laying out some basic considerations for approaching this subject, the chapter explores several concrete cases. How should a person decide whether to pursue a treatment that has very low probability of success when there are no other treatment options? Is it ever morally proper to forgo life-sustaining treatment for a chronic illness because the treatment itself is so burdensome? What are our moral obligations toward people in a persistent vegetative state (PVS)?

There are many other interesting and challenging bioethical issues that I do not address, of course, including middle-of-life issues such as cosmetic surgery, performance enhancing drugs, anti-depressant medication, and eating habits. This book, however, by setting forth the theological and moral foundations for bioethics and examining many of the most common and controversial bioethical issues of the present day, aims to provide Christians with a guide for difficult decision making that will equip them for faithful service to God in all matters of health and illness and life and death.

PART 1

FOUNDATIONS
OF BIOETHICS

Like all other people, Christians get sick and injured, deal with physicians and insurance companies, and confront death and dying. As they do so, Christians face bioethical issues not as machine-like decision makers but as individuals with personal histories, as members of various communities (such as families, churches, and nations), and as religious believers with certain convictions about God, this world, and the way that they ought to conduct themselves. Those histories, communities, and convictions will play a profound role in the way that Christians make their decisions when they face bioethical crises—whether they realize it or not. What does a Christian think about his place in the world, including the health-care maze? What does a Christian believe about God's sovereignty, the image of God, and human suffering? What virtues is a Christian pursuing as she grows in the grace of Christ by his Spirit?

Part 1 explores foundational issues such as these in order to make us better equipped to deal with the concrete bioethical issues discussed in parts 2 and 3. In chapter 1 we consider the Christian's relationship to this world and to the medical system. Believers ought to have a distinct perspective on bioethics in light of their Christian faith, and yet they continue to have responsibilities to participate in the bioethical debates and medical care of the broader world. Chapter 2 presents a number of important theological doctrines that are crucial for the Christian's bioethical decision making, including divine providence, the image of God, the nature of death, and the challenge of suffering. Finally, in chapter 3 we consider a number of virtues to which Scripture calls Christians and which form Christians into the sort of people who can live, suffer, recover, and die well.

1

CHRISTIANITY AND HEALTH CARE IN A FALLEN WORLD

This book focuses primarily on personal bioethical decisions that Christians must make for themselves or for loved ones. As such it does not focus on bioethics in the public square, that is, upon the economic, legal, and political dimensions of bioethics. The fact that the book has this particular focus, however, does not imply that the public dimensions of bioethics are unimportant or that Christians should be uninvolved with them. If I am to set forth a Christian view of bioethics, then I must provide at least a general perspective on the relationship between the believer's Christian commitment and his life in the broader—and largely unbelieving—world of health care. This is because thoughtful Christians who seek to be faithful in their private bioethical decisions will necessarily confront important issues that involve the public dimension of bioethics. Should Christians participate in the mainstream health-care system or should they establish their own Christian hospitals, medical schools, and insurance companies? Are Christians' biblically shaped convictions on matters such as abortion or euthanasia unique to Christianity, or are they also binding upon non-Christians? Are believers able to have morally meaningful discussions with unbelievers and, if so, how should these discussions take place?

In this chapter I argue that, though readers should strive to attain a perspective on bioethics and to make private health-care decisions in ways that are consistent with their distinctive Christian life (the focus of this book), they should do so while continuing to participate in the mainstream health-care system and making appropriate contributions to public policy debates about bioethics.

Christian Bioethics and Secular Bioethics: Contemporary Approaches

To describe important contemporary perspectives on the relationship of Christianity to the public dimensions of bioethics, I use the terms *Christian bioethics* and *secular bioethics*. By "secular" bioethics I do not mean "evil" or "godless" bioethics, but simply the discussions and debates about bioethics that take place in the broader world where there is no universally shared religious faith. Where do Christians stand in relation to the broader world of health care, and how should they participate in the bioethical debates that take place within this world? Bioethicists from a variety of theological and philosophical persuasions have attempted to answer such questions, with a remarkable divergence of opinion.

Five general approaches to the relationship of Christian bioethics and secular bioethics can be found among contemporary writers: (1) *secular bioethics only*, (2) *Christian bioethics only*, (3) *secular and Christian bioethics identical*, (4) *secular and Christian bioethics radically different*, and (5) *secular and Christian bioethics distinct but legitimate*.

Secular Bioethics Only

Writers who represent the first category, *secular bioethics only*, make morally serious arguments about bioethical issues for society as a whole and do so through philosophical or pragmatic argumentation. Though some of these bioethicists are religious people, their writings are nontheological, and they seek to address all people in a way that appeals to their moral sensibilities no matter what their religious convictions. The influential framework for bioethics espoused by Tom Beauchamp and James Childress, often called *principlism*, falls into this category. Beauchamp and Childress argue for the existence of a "common morality" that is shared by all morally serious people in all cultures. This common morality is not a theory of ethics but a set of principles and norms of conduct. Beauchamp and Childress acknowledge that there are also moralities specific to particular communities and that some people in all cultures refuse to live by aspects of the common morality, but they believe that the common morality provides a means for cross-cultural critique of immoral practices in particular communities. Beauchamp and Childress derive four fundamental principles from the common morality that ought to guide the professional ethics of health-care providers: respect for autonomy, nonmalificence, beneficence, and justice. Through application of these principles in concrete circumstances, Beauchamp and Childress aim to provide an ethical standard for medical practice in a health-care system that encompasses people from a range of communities and creeds.

Another example of a *secular bioethics only* approach is that of Robert Veatch. Veatch argues against a medical ethics derived solely from within the medical profession and advocates instead a medical ethics that emerges out of a social contract or covenant among all the members of society—medical professionals and nonprofessionals, those with social power and those without it. Though Veatch determines the content of bioethics in a way different from Beauchamp and Childress, the two approaches agree in seeking to develop a universally applicable bioethics governing a medical system comprised of people from all communities and faiths.

Christian Bioethics Only
A starkly different alternative to the *secular bioethics only* perspective is the *Christian bioethics only* approach. Adherents to this approach set forth a bioethics derived solely from their theological convictions and wish their distinctively Christian approach to bioethics to control all health-care practice. John Frame's *Medical Ethics* provides an example. Appealing to the doctrine of *sola Scriptura*, Frame sets out to answer various bioethical questions through application of biblical teaching. He notes the deficiencies of secular bioethics, but never discusses whether secular bioethics is a legitimate enterprise in any respect, nor does he acknowledge the legitimacy or usefulness of any nonbiblical source of moral knowledge (such as a concept of natural law known through God's general revelation). For Frame, society-wide bioethical questions are simply to be solved by applying biblical principles. Should the child of a Jehovah's Witness be given a blood transfusion against the wishes of her parents? Frame states

that the Bible considers people "competent" who obey God's will, and therefore since Jehovah's Witnesses have a false view of God, they are not competent to make such decisions for their children. Civil courts should order the transfusion against their objections. What if a physician becomes concerned about the question of confidentiality? Frame says that he should require his patients to agree to "biblical principles of confidentiality."

Other examples of a *Christian bioethics only* approach may be found in various visions of the Christian transformation of modern health care. Marsha Fowler's contribution to a volume of essays on Christian engagement in society's bioethical debates is illustrative. Appealing to the convictions of her own denomination (Presbyterian Church [USA]) and to her interpretation of the broader Reformed tradition, Fowler argues that the church is to be actively involved in transforming the health-care practices of the world. The church should have a prophetic voice in society and engage in political action and critique. Through an "incarnational ministry" that "embraces the whole of life," the church must seek to usher in the biblical vision of *shalom*. As an example she points to her own congregation's "health ministry," which offers aerobics classes, walking groups, and free blood pressure screening for church members and the community.

Secular and Christian Bioethics Identical

A third general approach is what I call the *secular and Christian bioethics identical* perspective. This approach differs from the *secular bioethics only* approach because it seeks to bring religious and theological considerations to bear upon bioethical discussions. It also differs from the *Christian bioethics only* approach in that it refuses to see theological reasoning as the only way to resolve bioethical questions and does not attempt to impose a distinctively Christian vision upon the broader society. This *secular and Christian bioethics identical* approach is probably best exemplified by a number of prominent Roman Catholic bioethicists. These writers refer to a concept of natural law in order to identify sets of goods, values, and experiences that are common to all people, promote general human flourishing, and provide a foundation for a universal and cross-cultural morality. Bioethics, then, ought to develop in conformity with this universal morality.

For such writers, Christianity and theological truth contribute little or nothing substantive to bioethics, but serve to reinforce and enrich natural law bioethics in various ways. For the late Richard McCormick, "the Christian tradition only illumines human values, supports them, provides a context for their reading at given points in history. It aids us in staying human by underlining the truly human against all cultural attempts to distort the human." For Lisa Sowle Cahill, theology can contribute to bioethics by raising awareness of the importance of justice and social solidarity and "explicitly religious narratives and symbols can also have a public role in widening the moral imaginations of people from diverse traditions and faiths." James Walter and Thomas Shannon argue that religion, and specifically their Roman Catholic tradition, illumines or "adds value to" certain aspects of issues that are often overlooked, such as inclusive concern for all people through ideas of the common good, justice, and human dignity. For all of these Roman Catholic ethicists, theology serves primarily to clarify, reinforce, and inspire adherence to truth about bioethics that is generally known and applicable to all people apart from Christian conviction.

Secular and Christian Bioethics Radically Different

Almost diametrically opposite this last perspective is the *secular and Christian bioethics radically different* approach. The most well-known advocate of such an approach is H. Tristram Engelhardt, a physician and philosopher who converted in mid-career to Eastern Orthodox Christianity. Engelhardt takes a very pessimistic view of the possibility of genuine moral discourse in a pluralistic secular society. In the post-Enlightenment world, Engelhardt argues, there are no commonly held metaphysical or theological convictions that could serve as a basis for substantive moral conversation and agreement. Some common, secular bioethics is possible, but it is *procedural* only, not substantive. In other words, secular bioethics is simply a set of procedures and rules that people agree to live by. This is what Engelhardt calls the "principle of permission" that binds people who are moral strangers to one another.

Yet Engelhardt also describes a Christian bioethics that is as substantively rich as secular bioethics is substantively poor. Engelhardt believes that traditional Christianity (particularly in its Eastern Orthodox expression), through its theological teaching about life, grace, and union with God, provides the basis for a profound bioethics that binds communities who adhere to these teachings. Hence Christian bioethics must be radically distinct from the secular bioethics that rests only upon the bare will of individuals consenting to live with one another in a certain way. Not surprisingly, Engelhardt encourages Christians to develop their own medical-care system in order to put into practice their distinctive moral convictions.

Secular Bioethics and Christian Bioethics Distinct but Legitimate

I label the final approach to these issues *secular bioethics and Christian bioethics distinct but legitimate*. Unlike the first two approaches, this approach seeks to account for both a Christian, theological inquiry into bioethics and a common, secular inquiry in which people from various religious convictions can participate. Unlike the *secular and Christian bioethics identical* approach, this approach does not simply equate secular and Christian bioethics, but recognizes that Christian bioethics rests on theological truths unknown to the broader world and hence cannot be substantively identical to secular bioethics. Finally, this approach differs from the *secular and Christian bioethics radically different* approach in believing that secular bioethics is not simply procedural but can involve genuine and meaningful moral discussion.

We find examples of the *distinct but legitimate* approach in both Roman Catholic and Protestant sources. Among Roman Catholics, for instance, Edmund Pellegrino and David Thomasma have written two books whose very titles hint at their approach: *The Virtues in Medical Practice* (1993) and *The Christian Virtues in Medical Practice* (1996). In the first volume, they use a philosophical conception of virtue in order to set forth an "internal morality of medicine" (i.e., a medical ethics derived from the goals that the practice of medicine seeks to attain, not a medical ethics derived from the principles of a general theory of ethics). In the second volume Pellegrino and Thomasma argue that these philosophical virtues, when combined with (Roman Catholic) Christian commitment, are transformed to a level of grace. Christian commitment brings "charity" into the picture. Charity gives new insight into the virtues and "perfects" philosophical morality through transcending the possibilities of nature. A Christian ethic of medicine, therefore, imposes obligations that are purely optional or supererogatory from a naturalistic perspective.

Among evangelical Protestants, John Jefferson Davis, Scott Rae, and Paul Cox offer examples of this *distinct but legitimate* approach but in a different vein from the Roman Catholic perspective of Pellegrino and Thomasma. These three evangelical writers believe that Christians must operate within the broader health-care system and participate in its bioethics debates, and they encourage Christians to utilize arguments from general revelation (or natural law) rather than exclusively from Scripture in order to be as persuasive as possible when dealing with unbelievers. Nevertheless, they also recognize that Christians' knowledge and experience of redemption in Christ, as revealed in Scripture, provides crucial perspective on bioethics that shapes a Christian approach to bioethics in significant ways. From a different angle, but also representing a *distinct but legitimate* approach, is the recent work of Joel Shuman and Brian Volck. These authors argue that modern medicine is among the "powers" ordained by God, but that it is also prone to abuse its power in god-like fashion. Therefore Shuman and Volck believe that Christians should continue to access the mainstream health-care system—with appropriate caution and detachment from its false promises. But Christians should also learn to care for one another holistically in the church through giving counsel to one another in their medical decisions, helping the poor to gain access to health care, and practicing hospitality.

Christianity, Secular Bioethics, and Mainstream Medicine: A Proposal

These few simple categories illustrate the variety of approaches to the question of Christian involvement in the health-care system and of Christian theological contribution to the bioethics enterprise. I believe that the most theologically sound and balanced approach is a version of the last: *secular bioethics and Christian bioethics are distinct but legitimate.* Christians should participate in the mainstream health-care system and contribute to its bioethical debates, while recognizing that their Christian faith has radically transformed their perspective on many important issues of life and death.

According to this approach, God has ordained a common cultural task for all human beings to pursue together, and the practice of medicine and the protection of life fall within this task. Christians may therefore participate freely in the secular health-care system with people of many different religious beliefs. The common cultural task, as God-ordained, is not morally neutral (even though it is not uniquely Christian), and thus Christians can pursue meaningful moral conversations with non-Christians in regard to bioethics in modern medicine. Within the context of this general, secular bioethics that concerns all people in their common life, Christians must also shape their individual and communal views of bioethics in accord with their distinctive theological convictions. The range of Christian truth about matters such as the image of God, suffering, death, and resurrection cannot help but mold their perspective on bioethics. Scripture's teaching should aid Christians in understanding the kind of bioethics that should govern all people in the public realm. But the knowledge and experience of God's grace in Christ should also instill a range of virtues and a perspective on life and death that will transform Christians' attitude toward bioethical issues and transform the way that they make decisions about a host of matters for which there are no universally binding moral rules.

The Christian's Identity in the World

God created human beings in his own image and likeness (Gen. 1:26–27). This rich theological truth, to be explored in more detail in the next chapter, is foundational for bioethics in establishing human beings as creatures of great dignity and honor, called to *life* and threatened with death only as a curse and punishment for disobedience to God. After the fall into sin, God placed this curse upon the human race and consigned human beings to return to the dust from which they were taken (Gen. 3:19). Alongside this curse came the first proclamation of the gospel, promising that a seed of the woman would crush the head of the serpent's seed (Gen. 3:15). The human race would be a divided race, therefore, comprised of those who cling by faith to this coming Savior and those who persist in rebellion against God. The early chapters of Genesis describe Cain and his progeny and the builders of the tower of Babel as examples of the latter group, but also point to Noah and Abraham as members of the remnant who worshiped the one true God and clung to his promises. God made a covenant with Abraham that set him and his family apart from the world yet promised that through him blessing would come to all the peoples of the earth. Augustine, in his famous *The City of God*, identified these two groups of human beings as constituting two cities that live in conflict and enmity with one another.

Augustine also noted that the people of these two cities mix in this world. Though the two cities have different destinies in the age to come, they live side by side here and now. Though God placed a curse on the human race, he did not let it sink into complete chaos. Many sorts of people—both believers and unbelievers—live law-abiding lives in society and make productive contributions to culture. This is evident in several ways already in Genesis 4. God put a "mark," or oath, upon Cain (Gen. 4:15) in order to indicate that a system of justice will exist on earth (however imperfectly). Cain went on to build a city (Gen. 4:17), and three of his descendents, Jabal, Jubal, and Tubal-Cain, became the fathers of three great areas of culture: agriculture, music, and metallurgy (Gen. 4:20–22). After the flood, God entered into a covenant with Noah and through him with "every living creature" (Gen. 9:10, 12, 15–16). This covenant made no promise of forgiveness of sins or eternal life, but did assure all creation that God would uphold the order of nature, that family life would continue, and that a human justice system would be operative (Gen. 8:22; 9:1, 5–7). Genesis 4:15 and 9:6 are particularly relevant. In both of these texts God ordained a system of human justice not as the sole possession of those who believed in him but as the common possession of the human race. In both texts the particular crime that prompts the need for justice is *murder*, the ultimate dishonoring of human *life*. Genesis 9:6 even reminds readers that God created man in his image:

> Whoever sheds man's blood,
> By man shall his blood be shed,
> For in the image of God
> He made man.

Protection of life in the human justice system takes place because of the enduring dignity and honor of human beings as the pinnacle of God's creation.

These opening chapters of Genesis, therefore, indicate that though God has called out a people for himself from the world and promised them salvation from their sins, he has also ordained that all people, whatever their religious convictions, must live together as divine image bearers entrusted with the continuing tasks of human culture: having children, building cities, planting farms, making music, forging metal, and especially securing justice against wrongdoers. Of course the religiously mixed societies of this world will often fail miserably at these tasks. Biblical accounts of the flood, Babel, and Sodom and Gomorrah testify about particularly egregious failures, and history is littered with stories of cultural perversions small and great. Yet cultural achievements and just judgments also fill the pages of history, and God's people have rightly participated in and benefited from this work. Though set apart unto salvation by a divine covenant, Abraham did not isolate himself from the world, but made covenants with its civil leaders (Gen. 21:27–34), participated in its commerce (Gen. 23:10–20), fought in its wars (Gen. 14:1–16), and engaged in meaningful moral discussions about questions of justice (Gen. 20:8–13). For a time, and for particular purposes in his larger plan of redemption (see Gal. 3:19–24), God set aside Old Testament Israel from the world in the promised land of Canaan. In the land, Israel was to continue pursuing basic human cultural pursuits such as childrearing, agriculture, music, and justice, though it did so not with the world but separated from the world. Even Old Testament Israel, however, exercised cultural camaraderie with foreigners and unbelievers *outside of the land* (e.g., 1 Kings 5:1–12), and this was particularly evident when they were exiled in Babylon (Jer. 29:4–9).

The New Testament instructs God's people to conduct themselves similarly to Abraham and the exiles in Babylon. The New Testament church is not like Old Testament Israel, an ethnically defined people living in one small geographical area, but is a multiethnic people residing throughout the world. Like Abraham, members of the New Testament church are pilgrims and sojourners in lands where they live side by side with those who do not know the one true God (Heb. 11:8–10, 13–16; 1 Pet. 1:1; 2:11). Significantly, Revelation 17–18 describes the church as living in *Babylon*, like the Jewish exiles of old. This Babylon, representing the cities of this world, is a place of commerce and cultural achievement. Its promises of wealth, honor, and security are deceptive and fleeting, and God warns believers to be on guard against its allures. Believers must be separate from the world in purity (2 Cor. 6:14–18), must be zealous for the holiness of the church (1 Corinthians 5), must strive to take every thought captive to Christ (2 Cor. 10:4–5), and must be transformed in the renewing of their minds (Rom. 12:2). In short, the ancient conflict of Genesis 3 between the seed of the serpent and the seed of the woman is alive and well, and Christians must be on guard against the assaults of Satan (1 Pet. 5:8). Yet this is not the entire story of the New Testament. Paul reminds his readers that though the church is to be a holy community, it is not called to leave the world, but must continue to associate with the wicked in their daily lives (1 Cor. 5:9–10). It will purchase and use the things of this world, though never becoming engrossed by them (1 Cor. 7:29–31). The civil authority that God implicitly gave to kings and governors in Genesis 4:15 and 9:6 still holds sway, and believers must submit to their work of bearing the sword for the enforcement of justice (Rom. 13:1–7). Though they are not *of* Babylon, they must continue for a time to live *in* Babylon and participate with unbelievers in a range of cultural pursuits.

This biblical overview of the relation of Christians to the broader culture is of the greatest relevance to questions about Christianity and bioethics. For one thing, Christians must be aware of the ongoing conflict between themselves and the seed of the serpent described in Genesis 3:15. Satan was a "murderer from the beginning" (John 8:44), and thus Christians should not be surprised to find the forces of a "culture of death" present in society. Believers must be vigilant and bear testimony in their evangelism and apologetics to the truth that is in Christ and to the value of life *over against* the spirit of the world.

Bioethics as a Common Task

In addition to this important task of bearing testimony for Christ over against the evil forces of this world, however, Christians have another crucial responsibility: pursuing medical progress and thinking morally about health care *alongside* and *in common with* this world. If *bio*ethics at the most general level concerns moral issues related to the protection and promotion of *life*, then Christians cannot treat bioethics as if it is their concern alone and as if they have a monopoly on thinking through bioethical problems. As noted above in relation to biblical texts such as Genesis 4:15, Genesis 9:6, and Romans 13:7, the protection of life is a task that God entrusts to the *whole human race* through its civil officials. By his own appointment, God calls Christians to protect human life and to promote its flourishing in concert with people who do not share their faith. If raising children, farming, making music, forging metal, and pursuing justice are common tasks, then the art of medicine must be too. As Christians and non-Christians alike study ways to make their crops grow better and to make their music more beautiful—and share the fruits of their learning with each other—so Christian and non-Christian researchers, physicians, and patients together should seek to care for the body and to heal its ills. When evil forces intervene and lovers of death undermine the value of human life, Christians alongside unbelievers are called to seek just resolutions.

For such reasons Christians have no compelling reason to abandon the mainstream health-care system or to seek medical care from Christians only. Community hospitals, medical schools, insurance companies, and medical practice groups are legitimate expressions of the common cultural task that God bestowed upon the human race as a whole. Immoral things happen within such institutions, of course. Within all cultural institutions people (sometimes professing Christians themselves) perpetrate terrible things, but this does not strip these institutions of their God-ordained legitimacy. The Roman government toward which Paul commanded obedience in Romans 13:1–7 was far more brutal than any contemporary Western government. The so-called culture of death is indeed at work in today's health-care establishment, but a culture of life is vibrantly present there as well. Today more than any other time in history the practice of medicine is able to alleviate pain, heal diseases, and hold death at bay. Many readers of this book would not have survived infancy had they been born two hundred years ago, and most of the others would have lived with severe discomfort that a simple trip to Walgreen's or the dentist can now easily cure. For Christians to cut themselves off from the amazing progress of modern medicine is to do disservice to the cause of life and its flourishing.

Likewise, Christians have good reason to participate in bioethics discussions and debates in the public square, and to do so in ways that respect the God-ordained character of its cultural life. Most bioethical issues are social and political issues in some respects. Society as a whole, and civil government in particular, is entrusted with the protection of life and the enforcement of justice against those who threaten it. Thus issues such as abortion, stem-cell research, fertility methods, and assisted suicide, insofar as they concern important and controversial questions of life and death, demand some sort of political resolution.

Political decision—by action or nonaction—must determine whether such practices are to be permitted or forbidden. Bioethical questions also arise in nonpolitical social settings such as hospitals and medical schools and in the development of professional responsibility codes for health-care workers. Christians and non-Christians alike have a stake in these debates, and Christians have no privileged place in the public square, the realm where God wills Christians and non-Christians to live in common. Thus Christians have an obligation to engage in these bioethics discussions in ways that respect the fact that the public square is meant for Christians and non-Christians together. To this extent Christians have an interest in "secular" bioethics.

This Christian interest in secular bioethics does not mean that believers are ever to give up their Christian presuppositions or to set aside Scripture as their highest authority. Christians' commitment to Scripture must define their views of human nature, suffering, death, and resurrection in ways that will always be determinative for their moral thinking. Yet since God has established civil society in its many dimensions as a common realm, believers cannot demand adherence to the Christian Scriptures as a condition for participating in debates in the public square. Christians may be grateful that God has revealed himself and his law in nature as well as in Scripture. This is often referred to as *natural revelation*. Scripture teaches that creation in general and the human conscience in particular make known to all human beings crucial things about God and his moral will for them (Ps. 19:1; Rom. 1:18–32; 2:14–15). By their nature as image bearers of God, all people know something of the value of human life and the need that it be protected (Gen. 9:6; Rom. 1:29). These same biblical texts remind us that unbelievers are prone to corrupt and to disobey the things that they know by nature. Yet they do *know* the moral law of God (Rom. 1:19–21, 32) and often *do* it (Rom. 2:14), albeit in an external and partial way.

For such reasons Christians can have genuine *moral* conversations with non-Christians. Secular bioethics can be bio*ethics*. Christians do not share basic presuppositions about God and this world with non-Christians (as a subjective matter), but God's natural revelation about himself and his world is common to them both (as an objective matter). While Christians must always look to Scripture to shape and correct their own understanding of natural revelation, creative appeal to the truths that unbelievers *know* by natural revelation provides a way for Christians to engage in meaningful moral conversations in the public square with those who do not acknowledge the authority of Scripture. While the ethics of Scripture specifically addresses people *as Christians*, those who have died and been raised with Christ, the moral law revealed in nature addresses all people *as human beings*. That is, Scripture commands obedience as a response to the redemption experienced in Christ while the moral law of nature places obligations upon all people based on their common created humanity. Natural revelation therefore provides an appropriate means for Christians to converse with non-Christians in the bioethics of the broader world.

Christians surely must be modest in their expectations about what can be accomplished in their participation in secular bioethics. They can be confident in God's promises to preserve this created world and its civil society until the end of history (Gen. 8:22) and thus that their participation in its life will not be in vain. But they should also be sober-minded in light of biblical assurance that the world will remain desperately sinful, full of suffering and persecution for Christians, until the end of history (e.g., 2 Thess. 1:5–10; 2 Tim. 3:1–5). Christian participation in secular bioethics, primarily through creative appeals to natural revelation, should never be tainted with utopian dreams. Secular bioethics will not usher in the righteousness of Christ's heavenly kingdom.

Christian participation in conversations in the public square should not be confused with the church's proclamation of the gospel and hope of everlasting life in a new heavens and a new earth. At best, Christian participation in the world's wrestling with bioethics questions is a means for God's gracious preservation of a measure of justice and well-being in this "present evil age" (Gal. 1:4). At certain times and places evil flourishes to a degree that leaves Christians with little opportunity to participate in the public square while maintaining their integrity and thus forces them to withdraw from public life and to pray for better days. It is hard to imagine, for example, how faithful Christians could meaningfully contribute to the public "bioethics" of Nazi Germany with its eugenics programs and its horrendous scientific experimentation on people deemed expendable. But ordinarily Christians are called to participation, to whatever extent is possible, albeit with modest expectations.

Conclusion

Christians should participate in the health-care system of the broader world and should contribute to public discussions of bioethics controversies in ways appropriate to the fact that the public square is divinely ordained as common space among believers and unbelievers. Much more could be said about strategies and arguments that Christians might employ as they interact with unbelievers about public bioethical issues. However, this book focuses on developing a distinctively Christian perspective on bioethics to equip believers for making personal decisions for themselves and their loved ones about health-care issues. Civil law and the medical system ought to recognize moral boundaries that seek to promote health and to protect life, and Christians must live within these boundaries. But within these boundaries, Christians also have the freedom to make many personal decisions about how they structure their lives in response to issues of health, illness, and death. As we make these decisions, we should recognize that the truths of the Christian faith have transformed our understanding of the meaning of earthly life, the significance of marrying and procreating, the purpose of suffering, and the process of dying. The next chapter begins to explain why that is the case.

2

THEOLOGICAL DOCTRINES

Bioethical dilemmas, both small and great, can only be resolved in the context of our ongoing call to know God, trust in Christ, and walk according to his Holy Spirit. The bioethical decisions that we make, therefore, ought to reflect a proper understanding of the truths and way of life revealed in Scripture. We must explore the theological doctrines and Christian virtues that define our faith and life generally, but that also have special importance for the challenges that arise from contemporary bioethics.

I will focus on four areas of theological doctrine in this chapter: the sovereignty of God and the nature of his providential governing of all human history; human nature, and especially the various aspects of bearing the image of God; the nature of death, both as it confronts all people and as it is radically transformed for the Christian by the life, death, and resurrection of Christ; and the nature and place of the suffering that every Christian must endure in the present life. These doctrines are crucial for the bioethical problems of the present day.

The Sovereignty of God and Divine Providence

When a serious illness or other health-related crisis afflicts someone, the first thing that she may find herself asking is, why me? This common response raises profound questions about the sovereignty of God and divine providence. Is God in control even over the powerful forces of disease and death? Is my illness really in accord with God's plan for my life? If God is sovereign over all things, how are the physical sufferings of his children compatible with his grace and love toward them? The doctrine of divine sovereignty can be an intimidating subject, but the bottom line is very good news: God is indeed sovereign, but his sovereignty always works for the good of his children.

Divine Sovereignty over Creation

Of all the remarkable things that Scripture tells us about God, perhaps none is as striking as its teaching that God is *sovereign*. The sovereignty of God refers to the idea that God not only knows all things comprehensively—past, present, and future—but also has planned and ordained all things such that everything, from the greatest events of history to the most obscure, comes to pass according to the counsel of his will. Scripture informs us that the sovereignty of God is a source of great *comfort and encouragement* for believers in Christ. Yet the doctrine of divine sovereignty is often subject to misunderstanding, and thus a careful consideration of what Scripture teaches is necessary. Perhaps no doctrine promises to shape our general attitude toward bioethics more profoundly than this one.

Scripture often speaks of God's sovereignty as extending to absolutely everything. God is the Creator, the one who called all things into existence out of nothing by a simple decree of his mouth (Gen. 1:1; Ps. 33:6; Heb. 11:3). This act of creation is precisely the reason why all things belong to him: "The earth is the LORD's and the fullness thereof, the world and those who dwell therein, for he has founded it upon the seas and established it upon the rivers" (Ps. 24:1–2). As human beings claim property rights in the things that they make, so God on a cosmic scale claims ownership over all his creation. This lordship over creation continues through the entire course of human history. By the prophet Isaiah, for example, the true God mocks the false gods of the nations who, unlike himself, have no comprehension of the past and no knowledge of the future, and can in fact do nothing to alter the shape of human affairs: "Let them bring them, and tell us what is to happen. Tell us the former things, what they are, that we may consider them, that we may know their outcome; or declare to us the things to come. Tell us what is to come hereafter, that we may know that you are gods; do good, or do harm, that we may be dismayed and terrified" (Isa. 41:22–23). In contrast, God proclaims through Isaiah that he both knows all things and is the one who brings all things to pass: "I am God, and there is no other; I am God, and there is none like me, declaring the end from the beginning and from ancient times things not yet done, saying, 'My counsel shall stand, and I will accomplish all my purpose'" (Isa. 46:9–10). This is true for events that we experience as good and those that we experience as ill: "I am the LORD, and there is no other. I form light and create darkness, I make well-being and create calamity. I am the LORD, who does all these things" (Isa. 45:6–7). What the Old Testament communicates with such eloquence the New Testament confirms with unmistakable clarity. The apostle Paul, for example, speaks of "the purpose of him who works all things according to the counsel of his will" (Eph. 1:11).

While these verses impress upon us God's sovereignty over every single thing in his creation, Scripture is particularly concerned with the sovereignty of God over *human* affairs. God reveals himself, in other words, as having special interest in presiding over the lives of his human creation. The psalmist, for example, reflecting on how God shaped him even in the womb, states: "Your eyes saw my unformed substance; in your book were written, every one of them, the days that were formed for me, when as yet there were none of them" (Ps. 139:16). This divine concern for determining the lives of human beings extends to both the things of greatest importance and those of seemingly little significance. On the one hand, God raises up and brings low nations and their rulers (Isa. 40:23; 45:13). He even chooses some individuals for eternal salvation, having mercy upon those whom he wishes and hardening others in their sin (Eph. 1:4, 11; Rom. 9:11–18). Yet this God who determines the grand things of this life and the next is also the God whose control extends to the minutiae that escape our own notice: "Are not two sparrows sold for a penny? And not one of them will fall to the ground apart from your Father. But even the hairs of your head are all numbered" (Matt. 10:29–30).

How does God exercise his sovereignty? Christian theology has often used the word *providence* to answer this question. Providence refers to God's sustaining all things in their existence as well as his governing and directing them to their appointed ends. Many of the verses previously quoted are commonly cited evidence of God's providential control over the course of history, but it may also be helpful to note that Scripture attributes a special role in providence to the Son of God: he "upholds the universe by the word of his power" (Heb. 1:3) and "in him all things hold together" (Col. 1:17). God himself, through his Son, upholds and governs all things, but he does not simply act directly and immediately upon creation, but often acts through intermediaries; that is, he uses the actions of his creatures to bring about his own will, even when those creatures have intentions that are completely different from his own. Joseph's brothers intended to harm him, but out of their actions God brought good for Joseph, his family, and even Egypt itself (Gen. 50:20). Later in the Old Testament God used hostile kingdoms to carry out his purposes for his people (Isa. 45:1–13; Hab. 1:5–11). Most remarkably, the hostile intentions of the Jews and Romans against Jesus were in fact God's way of accomplishing his ordained purposes: "In this city there were gathered together against your holy servant Jesus, whom you anointed, both Herod and Pontius Pilate, along with the Gentiles and the peoples of Israel, to do whatever your hand and your plan had predestined to take place" (Acts 4:27–28).

The Goodness of God and Human Responsibility

These biblical assertions of God's sovereign control over all things raise many questions, particularly how and why a holy and good God ordains so many evil things to happen and whether we are really responsible for our actions. Such matters often press themselves upon us in poignant ways in the midst of the situations that call for bioethical decisions. Infertility, illness, and the approach of death provoke questions about how and why God wills that we suffer. Wrestling with such questions can be extraordinarily difficult, and the answers are shrouded in mystery. Yet Scripture provides some important guidelines for coming to grips with these issues.

First, Scripture emphasizes that God is holy and righteous and that his sovereignty over all things does not make him the author of evil. Throughout Scripture God reveals himself as pure and set apart from sin. The evil things in this world indeed transpire according to the purpose and council of God. Yet the evil things come to pass in a different way from the good things, and the evil things bear a different relation to God's will. Some theologians have tried to capture this point by explaining that while God wills good things unequivocally, he wills evil things only by way of permission. In other words, though

God, according to his own wise purpose, permits evil to occur, he is not an evildoer. The apostle James writes, for example: "Let no one say when he is tempted, 'I am being tempted by God,' for God cannot be tempted with evil, and he himself tempts no one. But each person is tempted when he is lured and enticed by his own desire" (James 1:13–14). In contrast, God does claim to be the origin of all good things. James thus says a few verses later: "Every good gift and every perfect gift is from above, coming down from the Father of lights with whom there is no variation or shadow due to change. Of his own will he brought us forth by the word of truth, that we should be a kind of firstfruits of his creatures" (James 1:17–18).

Second, all human beings are accountable for their moral conduct (Rom. 1:18–3:20). God is sovereign, and all things happen according to the counsel of his will, so can God really blame us for what we do? Are we not simply carrying out God's will? Paul knew that such questions were bound to arise. Immediately after asserting God's sovereignty by saying, "He has mercy on whomever he wills, and he hardens whomever he wills" (Rom. 9:18), Paul anticipates the natural reaction: "You will say to me then, 'Why does he still find fault? For who can resist his will?'" (Rom. 9:19). Paul neither tells the questioner that he has a good point nor retracts his claims about divine sovereignty. He simply rebukes him for his defiant question: "But who are you, O man, to answer back to God? Will what is molded say to its molder, 'Why have you made me like this?' Has the potter no right over the clay, to make out of the same lump one vessel for honored use and another for dishonorable use?" (Rom. 9:20–21). Following the pattern of Adam (Gen. 3:12), sinful people try to shift the blame from themselves to someone else and even to God himself. The whole of Scripture proclaims that all people are accountable before God, however, and no appeal to God's sovereignty can contradict that truth.

These words of Paul's in Romans 9 suggest a helpful point: the relationship of God's holiness to his sovereignty over evil is a great mystery, as is the relationship of divine sovereignty to human responsibility. When Paul anticipates the objection that divine sovereignty cancels out human responsibility, he does not provide a philosophical explanation for their compatibility. Both doctrines—divine sovereignty and human responsibility—are true, and the Christian is to believe both doctrines even without a philosophical explanation. A similar dynamic appears in Job, which raises the question of God's relationship to evil so relentlessly. Toward the end of this book, God appears and speaks at great length, but he provides no philosophical explanation in defense of his ways. God simply reminds Job again and again of his own greatness and of Job's own smallness. Job's response is the proper one. He humbles himself and receives God's answer in faith, demanding no more explanation (Job 42:1–6).

This state of affairs should not surprise us or shake us (though it may humble us). If God is indeed sovereign over all things—knowing all things comprehensively and ordaining all of history in its tiniest detail—then it is not surprising to discover that there are things about God that transcend our small, finite understanding. According to Christian theology, the finite cannot comprehend the infinite. If God is sovereign, then surely he is mighty enough to make human responsibility a reality without compromising his own lordship. If he is sovereign, then surely he is mighty enough to bend the purposes of evil to his own purposes without thereby being corrupted by it.

When contemplating these matters, probably no passage of Scripture is more helpful to recall than Deuteronomy 29:29: "The secret things belong to the LORD our God, but the things that are revealed belong to us and to our children forever, that we may do all the words of this law." There are two sorts of things: those that are secret and those that are revealed. Those things that are revealed (such as divine sovereignty, divine holiness, and human responsibility) are to be believed, while those things that remain secret (such as the relationship of divine sovereignty to divine holiness and human responsibility), we are to leave in the hands of God.

The Benevolence of God's Providence

Before leaving this subject, it is good to remember a few more things that are revealed (not secret), things that will prove to be of comfort as we take up specific matters of bioethics. One of these things to remember is that God's sovereignty *always* works for the *benefit* of his people. If we were simply informed that God is sovereign over all things, we would not know whether to be encouraged or discouraged by this. We might suspect, in fact, that divine sovereignty is a frightening thing, leaving us no room to hide from an all-knowing God who searches the recesses of our sinful hearts. In the midst of his own severe sufferings, Job often felt this way, pleading with God to give him space and to leave him alone for a while. But in light of God's grace in Christ, Paul assures us: "And we know that for those who love God all things work together for good, for those who are called according to his purpose" (Rom. 8:28). God's sovereignty works for the believer's benefit. The resurrected Christ has dominion over all things now *for the sake of the church* (Eph. 1:22). God's promise, "I will never leave you nor forsake you" is meant for our encouragement, and prompts the response of faith: "The Lord is my helper; I will not fear; what can man do to me?" (Heb. 13:5–6).

A second and related truth that is revealed, and not secret, is that though we may face dire suffering in this life, God will never let his people be overwhelmed and consumed by it. God does not tempt us, and the temptations that he permits are never greater than we can bear. Paul's words are of great comfort: "No temptation has overtaken you that is not common to man. God is faithful, and he will not let you be tempted beyond your ability, but with the temptation he will also provide the way of escape, that you may be able to endure it" (1 Cor. 10:13). Precisely because he is sovereign, God is able to keep circumstances in check and to keep Satan at bay so that his people may persevere even through profound hardship and turmoil.

People in the clutches of illness or in the throes of death often feel a deep sense of helplessness and a fear of life spinning out of their control. Crises of health expose our human frailty in startling ways. But in the face of anxiety and despair, the biblical doctrine of God's *wise* and *benevolent* providence toward his people should be of the greatest encouragement. When our own lack of control is most clearly exposed, the assurance that God is in total control is wonderfully encouraging news.

Human Nature and the Image of God

Having reflected upon the nature and work of God, we now move to consider the nature of man, God's human creation. Bioethical debates are filled with questions about human nature. Controversies about whether embryos and fetuses have a right to life often turn on the question of what it means to be a human person and when person-hood begins. Debates about euthanasia frequently raise the issue of whether human life continues to have meaning and purpose when a person has ceased being able to enjoy and participate in ordinary human activities. Probably the most memorable and important way in which Scripture describes human nature is by calling us the image and likeness of God. Scripture uses this language in the very first verses that refer to human beings (Gen. 1:26–27). Many subsequent passages, in a variety of contexts, either refer to us as image bearers or allude to this fact. Our creation in the image of God is thus a rich subject that promises to have many implications for bioethics. There are several aspects of the image of God that are relevant to bioethical questions.

Destined for Life

One important aspect of the image of God is that we human beings are *destined for life*. God reveals himself many times in Scripture as the *living* God, and his image bearers were created to live. At first glance this may not seem very impressive. We speak of plants and trees and animals as living creatures, and thus life itself is not unique to human beings. But the sort of life that we enjoy as image bearers, despite obvious similarities to the animal world, sets us apart in many important ways. Initially we might think of the various attributes of the image described in Scripture. In Ephesians 4:24 Paul refers to the "likeness of God" as consisting in "true righteousness and holiness." This means that as image bearers we are *morally responsible* creatures, not driven by mere instinct, but created to live as holy and righteous persons (and thus only image bearers are really capable of being *sinners*). The living God is a morally responsible being, and so are we. Colossians 3:10 associates the "image of its creator" with "knowledge." The image of God, therefore, also means that we are *rational and intelligent* creatures. The living God is omniscient (that is, all-knowing) and supremely wise, and he created his image bearers, alone among his creatures, to live lives of intelligence and wisdom.

The life to which we are called as image bearers, however, is not simply about possessing certain attributes, such as morality and rationality. God calls his image bearers to put their moral and rational capabilities into action. The image of God is not static but active. From the outset of Scripture God reveals himself as active and productive. He calls things into being, he makes separation between things, he names his creatures, he commands them how to function, and he proclaims his creation "very good." God reveals himself as a king, as a royal and judicial figure who rules over his handiwork with wisdom, justice, and power. What does this imply about human beings? In Genesis 1:26, immediately after God says, "Let us make man in our image, after our likeness," he declares: "And let them have dominion over the fish of the sea and over the birds of the heavens and over the livestock and over all the earth and over every creeping thing that creeps on the earth." God had exercised supreme dominion over creation in the six days of Genesis 1, so it should come as no surprise that those who bear his image and likeness are called to exercise dominion under him. Like God (though on a much smaller scale), they are to fill the earth and subdue it (Gen. 1:28), they are to give names to creatures (2:19–20), and they are to make judgments about what is good (and bad) (2:16–17). Being image bearers of *this* God revealed in Genesis 1 means pursuing an active and productive life of benevolent dominion over the earth.

The life to which God calls human beings as his image bearers is therefore strikingly unique among earthly creatures: it is a life of intelligence and moral responsibility to be exercised as rulers of this world under God. God calls us to life, however, not only in this world but also in the world to come. We were destined not merely for earthly life but also for *eschatological* life, life beyond the confines of this present age. Christian thinkers through the centuries—from Augustine in the early church to Thomas Aquinas and Dante in the Middle Ages to a host of Protestant writers in the Reformation and beyond—have taught that if Adam and Eve had passed their probationary period in the garden, then God would have brought them and their descendants, with glorified bodies and without death, into a new heavens and a new earth. In other words, the everlasting heavenly kingdom to which we as Christians now aspire by faith in Christ would have belonged to the human race if our first parents had obeyed God's commands.

The opening chapters of Genesis do not communicate this idea explicitly, but a number of biblical considerations point to its truth. In Genesis 1–2, for example, God not only exercised dominion on this earth but also rested from his labors, a rest which Hebrews 4:1–11 explains is the heavenly Sabbath rest that Christians are now invited to share with God. Evidently God created man to image him in both his work (on this earth) and in his rest (in the age to come). The presence of the tree of *life* in the garden of Eden is also instructive. Though Genesis 2 introduces this tree rather mysteriously, we come to learn, after the fall into sin, that this tree concerned not temporal life but living "forever" (Gen. 3:22). Later biblical teaching more clearly reveals its true meaning: it is a tree of *eschatological* life, a pledge of blessedness in the age to come. Revelation 2:7 locates the tree of life in "the paradise of God" and promises its fruit to those who overcome the trials of this age. Later, Revelation 22:2 locates the tree in "the city," which refers to "the holy city, new Jerusalem, coming down out of heaven from God . . ." (21:2). Thus the life that the tree of life offers is life in the age to come, and this life was held out to Adam even from the beginning.

Romans 3:23 is also relevant: "All have sinned and fall short of the glory of God." Through their sin, human beings have not simply earned a sentence of death, but have forfeited enjoyment of God's glory. What is this glory which we failed to attain? Paul explains in Romans that "glory" is precisely the state of life in the age to come. He considers "that the sufferings of this present time are not worth comparing with the glory that is to be revealed to us" (Rom. 8:18). This eschatological glory, then, is what we forfeited by our sin and thus must have been within the reach of our first parents. Hebrews 2:5–10 also sheds light on man's original destiny. The author begins: "Now it was not to angels that God subjected the world to come, of which we are speaking." If not to angels, then to whom? The following verses quote from Psalm 8 and identify *human beings* as the answer: "What is *man*, that you are mindful of him. . . . You have crowned him with glory and honor, putting everything in subjection under his feet." It is important to recognize here that man *as originally created* was destined to rule the age to come. The author of Hebrews explains that we do not see this destiny fulfilled in human beings now, thanks to sin, but we do see Jesus, who as a true human being came to suffer in our lowly condition, but has been raised to glory and honor, and thus we ourselves are now called again to attain glory through him (Heb. 2:9–10). Jesus, as a true human being, fulfills the destiny of the human race in the original creation, namely, the destiny of enjoying dominion over the world to come with all glory and honor.

Human beings, therefore, as created in the image of God, were destined for *life*, even for *eschatological life*. When thinking about controversial bioethical questions, such as protection of human embryos and euthanasia, Christians often identify themselves as "pro-life" and their views as honoring the "sanctity of life." To assert that image bearers are created in the image of God is certainly to affirm that life is something to support and to honor. But we should always remember, whether thinking about the creation, preservation, or end of life, that the true image-bearing life to which all of us are called is one that far transcends temporal life here on earth in this present age.

The life to which image bearers are called reminds us of another reality. If we human beings were created to share in God's own glorious Sabbath rest, and to have the age to come subjected to us, then should we not be struck by the amazing honor and dignity of man? A human being is a person created to rule, in this age and the age to come. Human beings are exalted far above all creatures of this earth, made "for a little while lower than the angels" (Heb. 2:7), yet created with the destiny of being greater than the angels in the eschatological kingdom of God. This gives a whole new significance to phrases like "human dignity," which are so easily thrown around in bioethics debates. As we consider the proper treatment of fellow human beings, we must keep in mind just how marvelous that dignity really is.

Human Beings as Social Creatures

Several other aspects of the image of God have important implications for bioethics. For example, image-bearing human beings are social creatures. Even many pagan philosophers, observing our tendency to live in community and the necessity of community for human survival, note that we are "social animals." Moral decisions in response to infertility have profound bearing upon the marital relationship. Debates about abortion test our views on what sorts of responsibilities we have toward one another. Decisions about whether to discontinue burdensome treatment for a life-threatening illness have serious repercussions for the patient's family. The doctor-patient relationship itself often raises difficult questions about our mutual obligations. Bioethical issues, in other words, are inseparable from our identity as social creatures.

The first biblical discussion of human creation in the image of God brings to light a striking fact: God made man in his image "male and female" (Gen. 1:27). That is, not male alone or female alone, but male and female together constitute the "man" created in God's image. Though Genesis 2 describes the separate creation of the first male and female, this chapter also clearly communicates what 1:27 suggests: God never intended that there be simply one human being or even simply male human beings. Instead, he willed the existence of multiple, nonidentical human beings. In light of the tasks that

God commanded the human race to perform, such as exercising dominion and being fruitful and multiplying, the importance of the multiplicity and variety of the human race is evident. Without male *and* female the human race could not carry on the task of childbearing. And without *many* human beings, with a variety of skills and talents, surely the exercise of dominion over the whole world would have been impossible. God is infinite and performs a dazzling array of deeds. The human race as a whole, as a multitude of people with a wide variety of abilities and skills, is a much richer manifestation of the image of God than any one human being could ever be.

This social dimension of image bearing also extends beyond the original creation. God re-creates people in his image—specifically, in the "image of his Son"—in order that Christ might be "the first-born among many brothers" (Rom. 8:29). Redeemed image bearers constitute a community and display the likeness of Christ only in communion with one another. This is true in regard to our future heavenly life, which Scripture describes as taking place in a kingdom or city: the kingdom of God, the New Jerusalem. This is also true in regard to the church here and now. The Lord Jesus Christ established the church, to which he entrusted the keys of the kingdom of heaven (Matt. 16:18–19). God has given gifts to the church, among which are pastors and teachers whom he has appointed to minister the Word for the building up of his people (Eph. 4:4–16). The nature and obligation of our various social relations have much bearing upon bioethical problems, such as those arising out of reproduction and the process of dying.

Body and Soul

Another aspect of human nature important for bioethics is that human beings are both body and soul. Bioethical crises most immediately raise questions about the body, but those who are fighting pain or other disability know how deeply physical hardship affects our whole person. On the one hand we strive to maintain the meaningfulness of life even as physical abilities decline, but on the other hand we dare not denigrate the body as if its well-being is insignificant. What does Christian theology teach about human nature in response to such bioethics issues?

Christianity has taught, in theory, that we can never be reduced to either body or soul alone, because each person exists in body and soul as a unified being. But theologians have struggled to uphold this insight consistently. Much of the Greek philosophical tradition tended to downplay the body as an inferior part of our being and to look at death as the soul's release from its imprisonment in the body. There was always too much counterevidence in Scripture—the doctrines of the incarnation and resurrection most importantly—for the church to adopt such a view, but for much of its history Christianity has had to fight against tendencies to devalue the body or to look upon the body as the special location of sinful desires. More recently the pendulum has swung in the opposite direction. Due to the influence of various materialistic philosophies, many today insist that all we are is the physical body. All the human functions that were traditionally ascribed to the soul, they claim, can be explained by physical processes that take place in the brain. In light of these pressures upon Christianity from both sides—to devalue the body or to treat it as the entirety of the human person—it is necessary to say a few words in defense of a biblically balanced position that recognizes the existence of both body and soul. There are even good reasons to conclude that both body and soul bear the image of God.

That human beings have souls that are immaterial and distinct from the body seems to be an obvious conclusion from a casual reading of the Bible. Scripture speaks innumerable times of the "soul" (or of the human "spirit," which is used interchangeably with "soul" in Scripture). Some modern writers, however, have tried to harmonize Christianity with modern scientific claims that the physical or material is all that we are. They offer alternative readings of these biblical passages in order to argue that references to the "soul" are not to a distinct, nonphysical aspect of human nature. Although there is no space here to investigate such claims thoroughly, I mention a few brief considerations in response.

First, the words that the biblical writers use throughout the New Testament for the human "soul" and "spirit" referred, in the Greek language, to an immaterial, nonphysical aspect of the human person. The New Testament authors use these words repeatedly and never question their ordinary meaning. In fact, at one point Paul even explains a truth about the Holy Spirit by reasoning from the common knowledge that people have about the human spirit (see 1 Cor. 2:11). Though the New Testament writers did challenge certain conceptions about human nature that were common in their own day, they never challenged the notion that human beings have immaterial souls. Second, the New Testament refers to the human soul or spirit on a number of occasions *in distinction from* the body. For example, Jesus said, "Do not fear those who kill the body but cannot kill the soul . . ." (Matt. 10:28), and James states, "As the body apart from the spirit is dead, so also faith apart from works is dead" (James 2:26). Third, Scripture teaches that human persons continue to exist between their bodily death and their resurrection. When mentioning this so-called "intermediate state," the New Testament consistently uses the terms "soul" and "spirit" to describe believers who have died and gone to be with Christ (e.g., Matt. 27:50; Luke 23:46; Heb. 12:23; Rev. 6:9–11), and on at least one occasion it specifically refers to their existence as nonbodily: "We would rather be away from the body and at home with the Lord" (2 Cor. 5:8).

If it must be proven that we have immaterial souls, it is hardly necessary to demonstrate that we have bodies. Many Christians through history, nevertheless, have found it hard to affirm that the body is truly important and necessary for human identity. A number of biblical considerations should keep us from doubting how essential the body is, but surely the most powerful reasons are the incarnation and the resurrection. The doctrine of the incarnation reminds us that the eternal Son of God became man, which meant taking on not only a human soul but also a human body. He assumed a human body so that he might save our bodies and not only our souls. The doctrine of the resurrection has a twofold significance. First, Christ's own resurrection testifies to something amazing about human embodiment, namely, that the eternal Son of God not only took on a human body for a brief earthly life but also bears a human body today and forevermore. If the Son of God is pleased to bear a physical body, then the body should not be despised! Second, our own resurrection—which the New Testament places at the center of our Christian hope—warns us against wondering whether some better, nonbodily future might await us. The reunion of our souls and bodies at the resurrection will not be a disappointment but a cause for great joy, because then we will be holistically restored human persons again in the blessedness of Christ's everlasting kingdom.

This positive view of the body presented in Scripture even suggests that we bear the image of God in our bodily nature. Many theologians have felt uncomfortable with this claim, since God himself does not have a body. They have pointed instead to the soul as the location of the image. Several biblical considerations point in a different direction, however. First, when Scripture describes human creation in the image of God, it informs us that God made "man," "male and female," in his image (Gen. 1:26–27). There is no indication here—or indeed elsewhere—that the image resides in one aspect of the person or another. Rather, the language is holistic: "man" is the image, not "the soul." Second, the various attributes that characterize the image, such as knowledge, righteousness, and holiness (Eph. 4:24; Col. 3:10), and the various tasks the image bearers were created to perform, such as multiplying and exercising dominion (Gen. 1:26, 28), engage both body and soul. Finally, although God does not have a physical body, he does reveal himself in visible, material ways. The God whom we image is the God who made the heavens to declare his glory (Ps. 19:1), who appeared in majestic glory to Israel in the pillar of cloud and fire, and who made himself visible *bodily* in the incarnation of the Lord Jesus Christ (Col. 2:9). Amazingly, to see Jesus is to see the Father (John 14:9). In light of this, it should not trouble us to believe that we image God in both soul and body.

The consequences of this dual, body-soul nature for bioethics are surely significant. For example, the fact that our bodies are an essential aspect of our nature means that physical pain and suffering are real, not to be downplayed or dismissed. What we suffer in the body is truly *our own* suffering. But the fact that we are both body and soul also reminds us that our present bodies, which suffer and die, are not all that there is. We do not treat the death of the body as the end, for at death the soul continues to live and at the resurrection our bodies will be raised up. Thus, we do not consider the suffering and death of the body unimportant nor do we consider them the end of the story. In facing specific bioethical issues, we must strive to keep this biblical balance in mind.

Sin and the Image of God

A final matter regarding the image of God concerns the effects of sin. Foundational texts for understanding the image appear in Genesis 1, before the fall into sin, and we may well wonder whether all of the wonderful features of the image of God really apply to fallen human beings. On the one hand, Scripture emphasizes the devastating effect of the fall on the image. To put it one way, we were created as image bearers for righteousness and knowledge—and yet now "none is righteous, no, not one; no one understands . . ." (Rom. 3:10–11). Thus the New Testament speaks of believers being restored or recreated in the image (see again Eph. 4:24 and Col. 3:10). On the other hand, though the image has been corrupted and skewed by sin, the image is not completely erased. Genesis 9:6 and James 3:9, for example, instruct us how to interact with other people—whether believers or not—in light of their identity as image bearers. All people retain a unique human dignity and are called to exercise distinct human tasks in this fallen world. However corrupted by sin we may be, we must continue to treat one another as image bearers, with all due respect and honor.

Death and Resurrection

Theological doctrines concerning matters of death and the new life received through Christ are crucial for our study of bioethics. As we previously considered, God created human beings for life, and the fact that we refer to *bio*ethics points us to the centrality of *life* for the present book. But death is the great enemy of life, and thus death looms large for the discipline of bioethics. What then is death? How does our faith in Christ affect our perspective on dying? What practical difference does faith make in how we make end-of-life bioethical decisions?

The Nature of Death

God created human beings for eschatological life, placing our first parents through a probationary period and promising life in the age to come as their reward. Human death was not the way things were supposed to be. But God threatened death if they disobeyed: "of the tree of the knowledge of good and evil you shall not eat, for in the day that you eat of it you shall surely die" (Gen. 2:17). Death came into the picture only as a curse, the consequence of rebellion. As Paul explains, death is "the wages of sin" (Rom. 6:23). When Christians consider the multitude of ethical issues revolving around death, therefore, they must never view humanity as *naturally* mortal. Human death is radically *unnatural*, a terrible, perverted state of affairs. Death is an enemy, indeed, the "last enemy" (1 Cor. 15:26). As I will discuss in a later chapter, many modern movements designed to help people and their families through the dying process seek to portray death as something perfectly natural, as something that can be accepted and peaceful if dealt with correctly. Yet without a message of salvation, death can never be tamed in such ways.

Biblically speaking, what is the nature of this death that confronts human beings as the great enemy of life? Death consists of at least four aspects. First is bodily death, or perhaps more precisely, the separation of body and soul that puts an end to earthly life. This sort of death is usually in view when the Bible mentions death and dying, including God's original warning to Adam that disobedience would bring death (Gen. 2:17). This is evident in the curse that God pronounced against Adam, which concludes: "for you are dust, and to dust you shall return" (Gen. 3:19). Second, Scripture also refers to death as a moral and spiritual reality: "You were dead in the trespasses and sins in which you once walked . . ." (Eph. 2:1–2). Third, the curse of death has brought us under the tyranny of Satan, as Paul's very next words in Ephesians demonstrate: we were dead in our trespasses and sins, "following the prince of the power of the air, the spirit that is now at work in the sons of disobedience" (Eph. 2:2). The Devil was the instrument for bringing the first sin into the world, and death's grip upon all human beings involves bondage to him. One New Testament writer even refers to Satan as "the one who has the power of death" (Heb. 2:14). We must remember, of course, that Satan has no ultimate control over death. God alone is sovereign, and Satan must answer to him, as illustrated by the striking events of Job 1:6–19, in which Satan brings about the death of Job's servants and children, but only with God's permission.

The fourth and final way in which Scripture describes death is eschatologically, as death in the age to come. Revelation 20 cryptically refers to it as "the second death." This eschatological death is death in its ultimate and most terrible sense. It entails consignment to hell, the "lake of fire" (Rev. 20:14–15), and "weeping and gnashing of teeth" (Matt. 8:12). Scripture repeatedly describes this fate as never-ending, involving "eternal punishment" (Matt. 25:46), "everlasting contempt" (Dan. 12:2), and "unquenchable fire" (Matt. 3:12). These are weighty matters to contemplate. Many unbelievers have attacked this doctrine as making God unjust or bloodthirsty, and even many Christian writers have tried to soften the doctrine in various ways. Though it is not my purpose here to defend in detail the justice of everlasting punishment, one matter is helpful to recall. From the beginning God made man for *eschatological life*. Human beings by nature were destined for existence in the age to come, for existence beyond the confines of the present world. If we, by sin, rejected the destiny of eschatological life, what is left for us but eschatological death?

These somber matters highlight why death cannot be glossed over as something natural and potentially peaceful if handled correctly. Though clearly different people go to their deaths in different states of mind, there can be no truly peaceful death if death is a curse, a realm of experience in which Satan exercises his tyranny, and a door to a far worse fate than anything that people know in this world. Yet there is an exception to this truth, an exception that is quite literally life-changing and death-transforming. The Christian proclamation about Christ and his gospel effects a radical change in how a person should think about and experience death.

The Death and Resurrection of Christ

The good news about Christ and his work is nothing less than a message that death has been conquered: "For God so loved the world, that he gave his only Son, that whoever believes in him should not perish but have *eternal life*" (John 3:16). Christ has reversed the curse of eschatological death so that eschatological life may now be ours by faith in him. To appreciate this we must contemplate first the amazing fact that Christ associated himself with human death. Of the four ways in which Scripture characterizes death, Christ experienced three of them quite literally. He did not experience the moral and spiritual death that Paul described as death in our "transgressions and sins," of course, though Christ did suffer the consequences of this death by undergoing its curse for our sake. Truly he was the "man of sorrows" (Isa. 53:3) throughout his earthly life and especially as he "bore our sins in his body on the tree" (1 Pet. 2:24).

In regard to death as the end of earthly life through the separation of soul and body, Scripture testifies that Christ passed through this ordeal on the cross. Luke records Jesus' last words, "Father, into your hands I commit my spirit" (Luke 23:46), and Matthew recounts that after his last cry he "yielded up his spirit" (Matt. 27:50). Jesus' soul and body were rent apart. The Gospel writers highlight that Jesus truly died in this sense when they narrate the piercing of his side (which issued both blood and water) and the burial of his lifeless body in a tomb. Jesus' burial, in fact, reminds us that Jesus experienced not only the moment of death but also the state of being dead, that is, the ongoing separation of body from soul. Joseph of Arimathea handled Jesus' inanimate body on earth, while simultaneously the penitent thief was with Jesus' human soul in paradise (Luke 23:43). Through all of this it is important to note that Jesus did not go through life approaching death as a Stoic seeking to remain indifferent in the face of suffering. On the contrary, Jesus' agony in the garden of Gethsemane, as he pleaded with his Father to spare him from death if there was any other way, displays that for Jesus death was neither natural nor peaceful (see also Heb. 5:7). Although Scripture tells us relatively little about Jesus' experience of Satan's evil schemes as "the one who holds the power of death," it does recount one extended period of Satan's temptations, and it indicates that Satan returned to harass Jesus repeatedly (see Luke 4:13).

Jesus suffered not only his own earthly death but also grief resulting from the death of a loved one. The sting of death involves not merely each person's own experience of death but one person's sorrow at the death of another. John 11 informs us that Jesus knew this grief as well. In a very short but profound verse, John 11:35, we learn that "Jesus wept" at the death of Lazarus his friend.

What about death as an eschatological reality? Jesus does not suffer the punishment of hell for time everlasting, but Scripture indicates that he experienced the equivalent of eschatological death. Jesus genuinely took our place, which was condemnation unto death in the age to come. Jesus died for us, on our behalf (Rom. 5:6, 8; Heb. 2:9), bearing our sin (Heb. 9:28; 1 Pet. 2:23–24) and curse (Gal. 3:13) and enduring the wrath of his Father (Rom. 3:25). Perhaps most striking is Jesus' cry from the cross, "My God, my God, why have you forsaken me?" (Mark 15:34). This divine abandonment and the absence of comfort describes exactly the nature of eschatological death in the life hereafter.

Christ's earthly ministry is summarized concisely yet comprehensively in Philippians 2:8, where Paul writes that he was "obedient unto death, even the death of the cross" (AT). Jesus' obedience involved keeping the commands of God—as Adam should have done from the beginning—and enduring the curse of sin due to Adam and all of his sinful descendants. Before we explore the consequences of this work for us, we must reflect upon the aftermath of Christ's death, for his death could hardly be good news if it was the end of the story. Philippians 2:9–11, in fact, proceeds to describe, in beautiful poetic fashion, the continuation of the story: "Therefore God has highly exalted him and bestowed on him the name that is above every name, so that at the name of Jesus every knee should bow, in heaven and on earth and under the earth, and every tongue confess that Jesus Christ is Lord, to the glory of God the Father." These wonderful words proclaim that following his death (and because of it!) Jesus received *life*—resurrected, glorified life for the age to come. Hebrews 2:5–9, furthermore, displays that Jesus, the last Adam (see 1 Cor. 15:45), has attained the destiny originally offered to the first Adam: ruling the age to come. It is true that we look at human beings today and do not see anything resembling this destiny (Heb. 2:8), "but we see him who for a little while was made lower than the angels, namely Jesus, crowned with glory and honor because of the suffering of death, so that by the grace of God he might taste death for everyone" (Heb. 2:9). Original human destiny of life in the age to come has been achieved in Jesus.

One aspect of this resurrected life of glory to which Christ was raised deserves special mention, in light of important matters we will yet explore. Christ's resurrection was his *justification*. He has passed through divine judgment once and for all. This idea may seem inappropriate to some readers, since so often we associate "justification" with the forgiveness of sins, for which Christ had no need. But the term "justification" simply refers to a judicial declaration that someone is righteous. For us sinners, this declaration of righteousness includes the forgiveness of sins, but even for us the heart of justification is not *only* removing our guilt but also crediting to us the righteous obedience of Christ (see Rom. 4:6; 5:18–19; Phil. 3:9). When we are justified, we do not stand before God in a neutral position (credited with neither sin nor righteousness), but as positively righteous (credited with Christ's own righteousness). And thus Christ, though he never sinned, could be justified—in the sense that he was *declared to be righteous*. It is helpful to note that the act of resurrection is itself an act of judgment. The Old Testament says relatively little about the hope of resurrection, but its most eloquent witness to this doctrine declares: "Many of those who sleep in the dust of the earth shall awake, some to everlasting life, and some to shame and everlasting contempt" (Dan. 12:2). Resurrection is either *unto life* or *unto shame and contempt*. To be resurrected is to pass through judgment into one's everlasting destiny. Thus it is no surprise to find the New Testament state that Christ, by his resurrection, "was declared to be the Son of

God in power according to the Spirit of holiness . . ." (Rom. 1:4). Of course he was the Son of God before this, but here he was *declared* the Son of God as the last Adam, the God-man, who had completed his earthly task and would reign as the righteous Son of God and Son of Man forever. Even more explicitly, 1 Timothy 3:16 speaks of Christ being "justified by the Spirit" (AT), which in context seems to refer to the resurrection. Christ now *lives*, and he lives in glory as one who has been declared righteous once and for all, on account of his perfect life and sacrificial death.

The Benefits of Christ's Death and Resurrection

Christ's death and resurrection have the most profound and blessed consequences for those who trust in him. Christ died for us (Rom. 5:6, 8), and we died with him (Rom. 6:8), and thus he shares with us and bestows upon us the benefits of his resurrection life. Among these many benefits is our own justification. We rightly associate Christ's death with our justification, for there his obedience and suffering on our behalf reached its climactic fulfillment. But Paul also reminds us that Christ was "raised for our justification" (Rom. 4:25). The same justifying verdict that Christ received in his own resurrection is now bestowed upon us when we believe in him. We are reckoned righteous despite the guilt of our sin because of Christ's righteousness displayed in his resurrection from the dead. Thus Paul, shortly thereafter, writes that in Christ's work we have received the "justification of life" (Rom. 5:18, AT). Our justification by faith, so intimately tied to Christ's resurrection, is a justification that bestows upon us a right to life, a guarantee of resurrected life, a share in Christ's own heavenly life. By calling Christ the "firstfruits of those who have fallen asleep" (1 Cor. 15:20), Paul assures believers that they too, without any doubt, will one day be raised up (see 1 Cor. 15:22–23).

Paul's reflections in Colossians 3:1–4 point not only to what is future (our bodily resurrection) but also to what we possess now, namely, life in heaven while we still dwell on earth: "If then you have been raised with Christ, seek the things that are above, where Christ is, seated at the right hand of God. Set your minds on things that are above, not on things that are on earth. For you have died, and your life is hidden with Christ in God. When Christ who is your life appears, then you also will appear with him in glory." The original goal held out to Adam, glorified life in the age to come, is not merely something that we look forward to in the future, but is something that the justified possess now by faith in Christ who lives in heaven for them.

One of the most encouraging benefits of Christ's suffering and exaltation is that he is our great High Priest in heaven, willing and able to aid us in our trials because he himself endured temptation and emerged victorious. Hebrews 2:17–18 explains: "He had to be made like his brothers in every respect, so that he might become a merciful and faithful high priest in the service of God, to make propitiation for the sins of the people. For because he himself has suffered when tempted, he is able to help those who are being tempted." This same author adds shortly thereafter: "We do not have a high priest who is unable to sympathize with our weaknesses, but one who in every respect has been tempted as we are, yet without sin. Let us then with confidence draw near to the throne of grace, that we may receive mercy and find grace to help in time of need" (Heb. 4:15–16). "Consequently, he is able to save to the uttermost those who draw near to God through him, since he always lives to make intercession for them" (Heb. 7:25). Because Jesus underwent the full range of human experience, suffering and being tempted to far greater lengths than any of us ever will, we may go to him in every trial and find him fully able to understand as well as powerful to help.

All of this means that death and dying have been radically transformed for the Christian. What could only be seen as a dreadful curse and a source of relentless despair apart from Christ has been placed in a whole new light because Christ has gone through death for us and has been raised to new life. To be sure, Christians continue to grieve in the face of death, but we do "not grieve as others do who have no hope" (1 Thess. 4:13), because "we believe that Jesus died and rose again . . ." (1 Thess. 4:14). What is death, apart from Christ, except the greatest display of God's displeasure with us? But those who die in Christ are the objects of his special, gracious attention: "Precious in the sight of the LORD is the death of his saints" (Ps. 116:15). What is death, apart from Christ, except the manifestation of divine curse? But those who die in Christ receive a deluge of divine blessing: "And I heard a voice from heaven saying, 'Write this: Blessed are the dead who die in the Lord from now on.' 'Blessed indeed,' says the Spirit, 'that they may rest from their labors, for their deeds follow them!'" (Rev. 14:13). Apart from Christ *anything* is better than death, that entryway to the lake of fire. But in Christ, Paul can even speak of death as *preferable* to the continuation of life, for death has become an entryway to the very presence of his Lord: "So we are always of good courage. We know that while we are at home in the body we are away from the Lord, for we walk by faith, not by sight. Yes, we are of good courage, and we would rather be away from the body and at home with the Lord" (2 Cor. 5:6–8); "For to me to live is Christ, and to die is gain. If I am to live in the flesh, that means fruitful labor for me. Yet which I shall choose I cannot tell. I am hard pressed between the two. My desire is to depart and be with Christ, for that is far better" (Phil. 1:21–23).

To die and to be with Christ—that is blessed and desirable. Yet far better is the coming day when Christ returns and reunites our souls and bodies in the resurrection. Thus we rejoice now in the life that we have with Christ in heaven, believing that one day we will dwell with him there with resurrected body. "Our citizenship is in heaven, and from it we await a Savior, the Lord Jesus Christ, who will transform our lowly body to be like his glorious body, by the power that enables him even to subject all things to himself" (Phil. 3:20–21). As Paul assured the Corinthian church, he knew "that he who raised the Lord Jesus will raise us also with Jesus and bring us with you into his presence" (2 Cor. 4:14).

We will later explore in greater detail the consequences of such a faith, but even this brief reflection is sufficient to indicate how different a perspective on death Christian conviction gives. Whether it is contemplating death from afar, mourning for a loved one, facing decisions about one's own treatment, or caring for a dying person unable to make her own decisions, the decisive transformation of death from a fearsome enemy to a vanquished foe puts death and dying in a whole new light. Because of Christ's resurrection and our justification, death no longer confronts us as a sign of our condemnation. Now we face death not as helpless victims but as hopeful pilgrims waiting for our Lord to bring death to its final end, when we can say with Paul, "'Death is swallowed up in victory.' O death, where is your victory? O death, where is your sting?" (1 Cor. 15:54–55).

Suffering

All difficult bioethical decisions involve suffering, whether matters of infertility or illness or the approach of death. A bioethical decision is not merely a response to a health-care crisis, but at the same time it is also a response to suffering and the temptations that suffering brings. It may have been more pleasant to end the chapter with the preceding paragraph, contemplating the hope of our resurrection in Christ, but it is difficult to understand suffering properly without the theological foundation discussed above. Hence I address suffering last, not because it is the high point of our theology, but because here at last we can make some theological sense of this universal human experience that so often perplexes us.

The Inevitability of Suffering

Suffering is inevitable in this life. For Christians the question is not really *whether* we will suffer but *how* we will suffer. In other words, will we suffer in a godly way or not? Of course it is much easier to write (and to read) about suffering than to undergo it, and suffering is often romanticized on the written page. As arduous as the actual experience of suffering is—and its hardship is never to be minimized—nevertheless it must be stated that suffering is inevitable in the present age and even necessary for the Christian. Part of this inevitability arises from the curse that God placed upon creation after the fall into sin. Genesis 3:16–19 decrees that human beings will suffer in the very activities for which they were created in Genesis 1 and 2, including the bioethically charged matter of childbearing. Leaders in the Christian community sometimes tell their followers that if they just have enough faith they can escape these sufferings. They promise healing from illnesses and success in life's endeavors. But such a message is a misreading of Scripture. Though it may give momentary encouragement, it does untold long-term damage. God does not promise to spare Christians from suffering in this life, but he does tell us comforting things about the nature and significance of our suffering.

That Christians will suffer in this world is a frequent theme in the New Testament. Paul sought to strengthen the fledgling believers in one of his missionary churches, for example, by "encouraging them to continue in the faith, and saying that through many tribulations we must enter the kingdom of God" (Acts 14:22). He reminded readers that they were heirs of God with Christ, "provided we suffer with him in order that we may also be glorified with him" (Rom. 8:17). Elsewhere Paul explicitly teaches that special afflictions await Christians in the form of persecution for the faith. Among his sobering reminders of this truth is 2 Timothy 3:12: "Indeed, all who desire to live a godly life in Christ Jesus will be persecuted." Christians can expect these sufferings to end one day, but when is that? After Paul speaks of the necessity of suffering with Christ in Romans 8:17, he goes on to point to the "redemption of our bodies"—the *resurrection*—as our hope, the time when our present sufferings will yield to glory (8:23–25). In his discussion of persecution for the sake of the kingdom in 2 Thessalonians 1:5–12, he points to the day "when the Lord Jesus is revealed from heaven with his mighty angels" to judge the world and to reveal himself to his saints. This is the time when his people will receive "relief" from their afflictions. In other words, Christians should expect to be delivered from the sufferings of this world *when Christ returns and raises the dead,* and only then.

How is this claim consistent with the fact that Jesus and his apostles did many miracles of healing? Two things should be kept in mind. First, these miracles were signs of the kingdom of heaven that Jesus proclaimed throughout his ministry (Matt. 4:23). Jesus performed them not in order to show us the regular course of events for subsequent human history but to provide an anticipatory glimpse of the power of God to be displayed on the last day when he will raise his people from the dead and restore them to himself, body and soul. Second, the ministry of the apostles was a unique and temporary gift of God for the establishment of the church in its infancy. The one church of Christ, made up of Jews and Gentiles together (Eph. 2:11–22), is "built on the foundation of the apostles and prophets" (2:20). Christ gave many gifts and powers to his apostles that were not meant to continue through the long history of the church. Miraculous healings (performed by Christ) are prominent in the Gospels, they are only occasional in Acts (performed by the apostles), and are almost entirely absent through the rest of the New Testament. The New Testament does command us to pray for each other and at one point promises healing for certain (unnamed) illnesses related to particular (unnamed) sins when the elders anoint the sick person and they pray in faith (see James 5:13–16). But Scripture offers no general guarantee to Christians that they will be healed of their maladies if they just pray in faith or seek help from a person with miraculous powers. To suggest otherwise is to set Christians up for disappointment and despair.

When Christians suffer, whether from illness, persecution, or any of the many other hardships of life, they must remember that their afflictions are under the watchful care of God's sovereign yet mysterious providence. God is indeed sovereign over all things, and he has holy and wise purposes in all that transpires, but that does not mean that we are able to understand those purposes. According to Deuteronomy 29:29, we must cling to the things that God reveals to us but also recognize that there are many secret things whose meaning God does not reveal.

There may be no time in life when this is more important to keep in mind than when we are suffering. The instinctive response of so many people under hardship is to ask, *why?* or *why me?* We are told that God is wise and loving, and yet it is often entirely unclear what purposes could be served by our own or others' turmoil. Our suffering, in fact, frequently seems like counterevidence to Christian teaching about God's love and wisdom. In the face of this, we do well to ask what God has revealed and what he has not. Quite simply, God has *not* revealed the precise purposes of our personal afflictions, whether in our own lives, in the lives of others, or in God's plan for history. It might even be accurate to say that God *has* revealed that the simplistic yet attractive answers that we invent are *not correct*. For example, the book of Job teaches that the attempt to interpret suffering as the proportional payback for personal sins is misguided. Job's three friends spoke inaccurately about God in linking Job's suffering to his individual transgressions (Job 42:7). God never gives Job an alternative explanation for why a given person suffers in the way that he does, but instead he reminds Job how great he himself is and how small Job is (Job 38–41). In other words, he showcases the limits of human understanding before the immense wisdom and power of God. Job was correct, over against his three friends, to reject the simplistic equation of individual suffering with individual sin. But God still needed to rebuke him for questioning his love and justice when he could not make sense of the afflictions that he endured. Just because we do not know the answers to everything does not mean that God does not know them.

God's Grace in Suffering

We must beware of demanding to know the things that God has chosen to keep secret, but we must also confidently affirm the things that he has revealed and that are of great comfort to us in times of suffering. God promises to work out all things for the good of those who love him (Rom. 8:28) and to provide his Spirit to pray with and for us when, in our weakness, we know not what to pray (Rom. 8:26). He promises never to leave us or forsake us (Heb. 13:5) and never to allow us to be tempted beyond what we can bear (1 Cor. 10:13). Furthermore, Scripture assures us that our sufferings are not just ordinary human sufferings, because we are suffering *with Christ*. As we suffer "with him" (Rom. 8:17) and God works out all things for our good (Rom. 8:28), we are being "conformed to the image of his Son" (Rom. 8:29). Christ himself suffered first and only then entered into his glory. Thus believers, in conformity to their Lord, are called to "share his sufferings" (Phil. 3:10) for a while before joining him in the glory of his kingdom. Peter adds: "But rejoice insofar as you share Christ's sufferings, that you may also rejoice and be glad when his glory is revealed" (1 Pet. 4:13). James also picks up on this paradoxical command to rejoice in the midst of suffering. He instructs us to see our suffering as a refining of our faith and as an instrument for making us mature in our Christian walk: "Count it all joy, my brothers, when you meet trials of various kinds, for you know that the testing of your faith produces steadfastness. And let steadfastness have its full effect, that you may be perfect and complete, lacking in nothing" (James 1:2–4). Later, James interprets the story of Job along these lines. The book of Job ends with an account of Job's progress in the faith (Job 42:1–6), and James sees here the "purpose of the Lord," which displays that he is "compassionate and merciful" (James 5:11).

We cannot know exactly how God is refining our faith and conforming us to the image of Christ through our sufferings. These things so often remain secret in the midst of hardship and even afterward. Yet because we know that Christ has suffered and risen to glory, and thereby has sanctified our suffering and made it a prelude to glory, we may trust that God is at work even in our struggles. Job and the Old Testament psalmists often asked *why?* in the face of affliction. In Christ's cross and resurrection God has provided an answer—not a philosophical answer meant to satisfy the curious intellect, but a religious answer meant to comfort us in a way much better than a philosophical answer ever could. The cross and resurrection proclaim that suffering and death, though not fully understood, have been defeated.

The Limits of Human Nature and Human Action

Before I conclude it may be helpful to make explicit something that has been an implicit theme throughout this chapter: human beings have been given a great deal of latitude to shape their conduct in this world, but only under definite constraints that God has placed upon them. By divine ordination, there are limits beyond which human beings are not meant to go. We make free moral decisions, but it is futile to lust after moral autonomy liberated from divine sovereignty.

This truth is inherent in the nature of the image of God. God created human beings with amazing capabilities meant to be developed and utilized in exercising dominion over this world. God formed the earth, yet delegated its cultivation to man. But man was not only to image God in this creative freedom but also to remember that he was only a vice-governor. He was no less than the image of God, but no more than that either. The original temptation struck right at this truth. The serpent enticed Eve with the prospect that she would "be like God" (Gen. 3:5)—not by cultivating the earth under God's authority but by asserting her own authority over against God. Sinful humanity has continued to display this same hubris, ever seeking to transcend its own boundaries and to usurp God's place: "Come, let us build ourselves a city and a tower with its top in the heavens . . ." (Gen. 11:4).

One of the prime occasions for fallen human beings to transcend their God-given limits is in matters of life and death. After the fall God placed his angel at the entrance to Eden guarding the way to the tree of life, "lest he reach out his hand and take also of the tree of life and eat, and live forever" (Gen. 3:22). God himself would provide a way for human beings to live forever in spite of his sin—through the Lord Jesus Christ—but they persist in seeking their own way to immortality. The quest to immortalize ourselves was reflected in the salute to ancient monarchs, "O king, live forever!" (Dan. 2:4; 3:9; 6:6). Too often it can become the subtle goal of modern medical technology. Today there is even a movement afoot referred to as "transhumanism," which seeks, through the power of genetic therapy, the enhancement of human nature itself in order to overcome its present constraints. From a Christian perspective, however, there is an idolatrous futility to such dreams. Modern medicine is a gift from God that can make this present life better, but it cannot transcend this life. We may seek to reduce suffering, but it is futile to claim a right to be free of suffering. We may seek to improve the quality of life and even to postpone death for a time, but in vain do we strive to postpone death forever.

Conclusion

We have explored only a few theological doctrines, yet they are doctrines of great importance for the Christian life in general and for bioethics in particular. If the goal of this book is to be accomplished— exploring bioethical issues not as isolated moral problems but in the context of broader Christian faith and life—we must know what we believe about God, ourselves, and our relationship to God in this world and the next. Building upon this foundational material, we will next investigate some key Christian virtues that correspond to Christian doctrine. Later we will explore how the doctrines and virtues that shape Christian faith and life come to concrete expression amidst the bioethical challenges of the contemporary world.

3

CHRISTIAN VIRTUES

Imagine two Christians who have recently been diagnosed with a life-threatening disease. They face a monumental choice: should they pursue the only treatment available, a treatment that offers a small chance of success but is extremely costly and inflicts severe physical side effects? They look to Scripture for an answer, but realize that it does not address their situation. So each makes a decision according to her best judgment—one chooses to pursue the treatment and the other chooses to forgo it. Why did they make their respective decisions? How can we evaluate their actions as *moral* choices?

The concept of *virtue* provides an illuminating answer to such questions. By *virtue* I refer to a character trait that orients or disposes a person to act in a good way. If we ask the first Christian why she chose to pursue the treatment, she might respond, "Because I care so much about my little children who need a mother, I'm willing to go through this terrible treatment to give myself a chance to survive." Her answer suggests that the virtue of *love* was compelling her to act as she did. If we ask the second Christian why she chose to forgo the treatment she might respond, "God has given me so many good things in my life, including the prospect now of dying peacefully with my family nearby, that I don't need to do something desperate to preserve my life a little longer." Her answer suggests that the virtue of *contentment* inclined her to make her choice.

On the other hand, moral decisions like these are usually complex. If we probe a little deeper, the first woman might also confess that she chose to pursue the treatment because she has doubts about what lies beyond the grave and finds little attraction about the prospect of heaven. In this case our moral evaluation of her choice would certainly change, for her *lack* of a virtue—the virtue of *hope*—has also motivated her action. The second woman might admit that part of her decision to forgo the treatment was driven by a powerful fear of enduring its side effects. In this case, too, the lack of a virtue—the virtue of *courage*—contributed to her decision.

We must give attention to the concept of virtue. A great many people who have written about ethics throughout history have recognized that a thorough account of the moral life requires consideration of more than just particular actions. *People* perform moral actions, and what kind of person an individual is has great bearing upon what sort of actions she performs. We expect certain people to act in certain ways, and we are surprised when they act otherwise. When someone we know as a woman of great self-control loses her temper, we say that she acted "out of character." If we are interested in helping an individual to perform morally good actions, we must also be interested in shaping that individual into the kind of person who is able to carry out those actions. In the past generation, both theologians and philosophers have shown renewed interest in the study of virtue after many years of neglect.

This book is primarily interested in actions rather than virtues. We are seeking to understand the challenges of contemporary bioethics and the way that Christians should conduct themselves in the face of these challenges. But if Christians are the wrong sort of people when a particular bioethical dilemma confronts them, then they are much less likely to respond in the right manner. If Christians wait until a crisis arises to show interest in the character traits necessary to deal with that crisis in a godly way, it is too late. The whole Christian life must be a process of striving after the virtues to which Scripture calls us. God indeed uses crises in order to build character, but he also builds character beforehand for the purpose of bringing us through crises. Here we are primarily concerned with the virtues that prepare us to respond in godly ways to the challenges of contemporary bioethics.

We should keep two things in mind. First, God the Holy Spirit is the one who sanctifies us, in conformity unto Christ; only the Spirit is able to change our sinful hearts (Rom. 8:4–13). Second, Scripture calls us to seek after holiness (Col. 3:5; 2 Cor. 7:1); God is pleased to sanctify us by his Spirit and Word as we struggle against sin and strive to obey his law.

The various Christian virtues are interrelated, and there is no particular order in which they must be considered. But we will look at several key virtues in a way that reflects the inner dynamic of the Christian life and therefore seeks to clarify the relation of each virtue to the others. By beginning with faith and then proceeding to hope—and through faith and hope to love, courage, and contentment—we will see what is distinctively Christian about these virtues and how much they depend upon the doctrines considered in chapter 2. We will also consider wisdom, another virtue that is crucial for making good decisions about bioethical issues.

Faith: The Fount of the Virtues

Classical Christian theology, picking up on Paul's words in 1 Corinthians 13:13, has identified faith, hope, and love as the principal theological or Christian virtues. One drawback of such a move is that we come to think of faith as simply one virtue among many. In Scripture, faith is unique. It is unique because it does something that no other virtue does and because it serves as the fount or source of all the other virtues. In short, faith alone looks outside of itself, trusts in another, and receives life and salvation as a free gift. This is why, according to Reformation theology as it recovered the teaching of Scripture, faith *alone* justifies as it receives and rests upon Christ. Yet this justifying faith is never alone, for genuine faith always produces the fruit of good works. All the other virtues and the actions that flow from them are the fruit of justifying faith. Without faith it is impossible to please God (Heb. 11:6), and anything not done by faith is sin (Rom. 14:23). True faith is manifest by its love and all other good works (Gal. 5:6; James 2:14–26). For the Christian, all bioethical decisions must be made and performed as the fruit of our faith in Christ.

In chapter 2 we explored two central truths of the Christian religion: the death and resurrection of Christ. When the accomplishment of redemption through these great acts is proclaimed in the gospel, the most basic response is faith. The Philippian jailer asked Paul what he must do to be saved, and Paul's answer was simple: "Believe in the Lord Jesus, and you will be saved . . ." (Acts 16:31). Though there are other necessary responses that the apostles identify in their preaching in Acts, such as repentance and baptism, the New Testament as a whole gives the priority to faith (without thereby downplaying the necessity of those other responses). All of salvation comes by faith, as the well-known words of Ephesians 2:8–9 relate: "For by grace you have been saved through faith. And this is not your own doing; it is the gift of God, not a result of works, so that no one may boast." The New Testament highlights justification by faith as central to the gospel, but in fact all of the benefits won for us by Christ come through faith, including adoption (Gal. 3:25–26) and sanctification (Acts 26:18). What is the nature of this faith by which we receive so many blessings? Why, of all the Christian virtues, is faith singled out in this way?

A proper conception of faith is crucial for understanding why faith is preeminent among the virtues. The traditional Roman Catholic emphasis is on faith as *knowledge*, or as a particular way of knowing. People come to know some things by their natural faculty of reason, but they can know other things only by supernatural revelation, and these latter things are known by faith. The Reformation understood faith in a different way. The Reformers did not deny that knowledge is an aspect of true faith, for of course faith must have cognizance of that in which it believes. But in addition to the intellectual aspects of faith sometimes called *notitia* (knowledge) and *assensus* (assent), they identified a third aspect that is in fact the heart of true faith, *fiducia* (trust). Faith is *trust* in Christ for justification and all the benefits of salvation. Sometimes the term "extraspective" is used to describe this faith. The person with faith looks outside of herself, forsaking any confidence in her own works and resting wholly on the work of another, the Lord Jesus Christ. This extraspective quality is what makes faith unique and distinguishes it from every other Christian virtue. Only faith looks outside of itself to receive the work of another as a free gift.

This dispute about the nature of faith between Rome and the Reformation was not a peripheral disagreement. Because Rome understood justification to be a process by which an individual becomes personally and increasingly holy, it insisted that faith (as knowledge) must be "formed" by love if it is to justify. On the other hand, because the

Reformation taught that justification is not a process of becoming personally holy but a once-for-all judicial act by which God declares a person righteous on the basis of the imputed (credited) righteousness of Christ, it insisted that faith *alone* justifies because trusting in Christ and thereby receiving his imputed righteousness is all that is necessary for justification.

One striking way in which Scripture highlights the uniqueness of faith is by the frequent contrast of faith and works (or faith and law). Among many examples (e.g., see Rom. 4:13–16; 9:32; 10:5–6; Gal. 2:16; 3:10–12; Eph. 2:8–9; Phil. 3:9), Romans 4:4–5 describes this contrast in a particularly striking way: "Now to the one who works, his wages are not counted as a gift but as his due. And to the one who does not work but believes in him who justifies the ungodly, his faith is counted as righteousness." In other words, there are two conceivable ways in which one might be justified—declared righteous—by God. A person might perform works (perfectly) and hence be able to claim the reward from God by way of obligation, as one who has earned it, like a worker who has fulfilled a contract with his employer. Or a person might have faith in the God who justifies the ungodly and hence receive justification as a gift. Paul, therefore, singles out faith in contrast to all of the good works that a person would have to perform perfectly in order to be justified by God "as his due."

As stated previously, this faith that alone justifies is unique in that it is *extraspective*: it looks outside of itself and trusts in another (Christ) to receive his righteousness as a gift. Throughout the New Testament, of course, the object of faith is Christ himself. Scripture tells us not to have a vague confidence that things will turn out okay, but to have faith *in Christ* (among many examples, see John 3:16; Acts 10:43; Rom. 3:22). This faith in Christ is such that he who has it throws off all confidence in himself and his own achievements so that he might attain the "righteousness of God" in Christ: "But whatever gain I had, I counted as loss for the sake of Christ. Indeed, I count everything as loss because of the surpassing worth of knowing Christ Jesus my Lord. For his sake I have suffered the loss of all things and count them as rubbish, in order that I may gain Christ and be found in him, not having a righteousness of my own that comes from the law, but that which comes through faith in Christ, the righteousness from God that depends on faith" (Phil. 3:7–9). Paul's looking away from himself and grasping the righteousness of Christ may truly be characterized as *trust* because it entails a confidence that the one in whom we believe will in fact do what he has promised. As Paul expresses elsewhere, "I know whom I have believed, and I am convinced that he is able to guard until that Day what has been entrusted to me" (2 Tim. 1:12). He enunciates the same sentiment in Romans 4 when he describes the experience of Abraham, to whom God had promised a son in his old age: "No distrust made him waver concerning the promise of God, but he grew strong in his faith as he gave glory to God, fully convinced that God was able to do what he had promised" (4:20–21). What is the result of this trust, this faith? Paul continues: "That is why his faith was 'counted to him as righteousness'" (4:22); that is, by this faith he was justified.

Thus, faith is trust because it relies upon the promises of God in Christ, which can never fail. According to these promises, God justifies those who believe, a fact that should grant believers supreme assurance. Justification means that God has pronounced us righteous before him once and for all, and nothing in heaven or on earth can reverse God's decree that is based upon the perfect work of his Son. "If God is for us, who can be against us? He who did not spare his own Son but gave him up for us all, how will he not also with him graciously give us all things? Who shall bring any charge against God's elect? It is God who justifies. Who is to condemn? Christ Jesus is the one who died—more than that, who was raised—who is at the right hand of God, who indeed is interceding for us. Who shall separate us from the love of Christ? . . . For I am sure that neither death nor life, nor angels nor rulers, nor things present nor things to come, nor powers, nor height nor depth, nor anything else in all creation, will be able to separate us from the love of God in Christ Jesus our Lord" (Rom. 8:31–39).

Justifying faith is indeed set apart from all other works and all other virtues. Though faith alone justifies, however, it does not wipe out the other virtues from our lives. Quite the contrary. The person with faith, having been justified once and for all before God, will not fail to bring forth the fruits of a godly life. The following virtues flow from faith as its fruit and are particularly relevant for bioethics.

Hope

Perhaps the virtue that most evidently flows from faith is hope. Faith and hope are so closely related that many people have a difficult time seeing the difference between them. Both of them concern things that cannot be seen here and now (see Rom. 8:24; 2 Cor. 5:7; Heb. 11:1), and both entail confidence rather than doubt. Their chief distinction, however, lies in faith's orientation to the present and hope's orientation to the future. Faith lays hold of the promises of God and receives justification now. Hope, in contrast, looks to the future and the promises of God yet to be received. It is because of the blessings that we possess *now* by *faith* that we have *hope* for the *future*. Thus hope is a fruit of faith.

A discussion of hope must begin with clarification of what the term means. This is an acute problem, because "hope" as ordinarily used in Scripture, as a Christian virtue, is considerably different from the way "hope" is used in common, everyday speech. This does not mean that we should never speak of hope in the common sense, but we should be attentive to the shift in meaning.

Three things seem to characterize hope as it is used in our common speech. First, hope is directed at something *desirable*. We do not profess to hope for something that we do not want. Second, hope concerns things that are *possible*. When a course of action or a goal no longer appears attainable, we say that there is "no hope." Finally, hope looks to obtain something that is *uncertain*. People do not express hope for something that they have no doubt they will soon obtain. Thus hope in colloquial speech is aimed at desirable things that are possible but uncertain. When people say, "I hope we win the game tomorrow" or "I hope that she'll recover from her illness," we assume that winning and recovery are what they wish to happen and are possible, but are not sure things. We would not expect to hear, "I hope we win our game tomorrow" from someone who has bet his life savings on a defeat (thus making victory undesirable), or who is a fan of a team that is completely outmatched (thus making victory impossible), or who is a fan of a team that is overwhelmingly dominant (thus making victory certain).

The New Testament, on occasion, uses "hope" to refer to what is desirable and possible but not certain. Paul speaks in this way to describe his earthly plans, when he relates where he intends to go or what he intends to do (e.g., Rom. 15:24; 1 Cor. 16:7). Sometimes Scripture indicates elsewhere that what Paul "hoped" would happen did not come to pass. On these occasions Paul speaks in a colloquial way, expressing his desire for things that, from the standpoint of limited earthly knowledge, he understood to be possible without being certain.

But the New Testament's commendation of hope as a virtue that Christians pursue and possess is different from this colloquial meaning in two important respects. Christian hope is primarily *eschatological* (that is, pertaining to things not of this world but of the age to come) and Christian hope is *certain* and *assured* (that is, the Christian does not hope for things that are merely possible). Hope takes on both of these characteristics because it flows from faith.

First, Christian hope is eschatological, looking to the things of the world to come rather than to those of the present world. We can begin to appreciate this aspect of hope by observing its *future-oriented* character. As Paul states in Romans 8:24–25, "Now hope that is seen is not hope. For who hopes for what he sees? But if we hope for what we do not see, we wait for it with patience." We must wait for what we hope for precisely because we would not *hope* for it if we already possessed and saw it. Of course, hoping for something in the future does not necessarily mean hoping for something in the age to come. Hope in our colloquial speech usually looks to something that is future, but nevertheless attainable in this life. The broader context of Paul's words in Romans 8, however, indicates that Paul has an eschatological future in mind as he exhorts us to hope: "And not only the creation, but we ourselves, who have the firstfruits of the Spirit, groan inwardly as we wait eagerly for adoption as sons, the redemption of our bodies. For in this hope we were saved . . ." (Rom. 8:23–24). The hope in which we were saved, the hope that sustains us in the midst of the suffering of this life, is the "redemption of our bodies," that is, our *resurrection*. As Paul makes clear a few verses earlier, the time at which we receive this "adoption," the "freedom of the glory of the children of God," is when creation is "set free from its bondage to corruption" (Rom. 8:21). On the last day, when Christ returns, when believers are raised up and the new heavens and new earth are ushered in (see also 2 Pet. 3:4–10), Christians will receive the object of their hope. The New Testament, and Paul in particular, emphasizes the resurrection as the focus of eschatological hope for the Christian. The apostles' preaching in the book of Acts provides ample illustration of this point (see Acts 2:26–27; 23:6; 24:15; 26:6–8; 28:17–20). For example, Paul speaks of "having a hope in God, which these men themselves accept, that there will be a resurrection of both the just and the unjust" (Acts 24:15).

In his epistles, every one of which mentions hope, Paul expresses the same idea. For Paul, *our own resurrection* is the immediate object of hope (see Rom. 8:20–25; 1 Cor. 15:19; 1 Thess. 4:13; see also 1 John 3:2–3). But it is important to note as well that *Christ's resurrection* provides the basis for looking in hope to our own resurrection (see 1 Cor. 15:20; Eph. 1:18–20; 1 Thess. 4:14; see also 1 Pet. 1:3, 21). Paul's reasoning is not difficult to decipher. Christ's resurrection was the firstfruits, and hence the guarantee, of our own resurrection (1 Cor. 15:22–23). Christ rose for our justification (Rom. 4:25), and we rose with him (Rom. 6:5; Col. 3:1).

In addition to the resurrection, the New Testament speaks of several other blessings of the age to come as the objects of our hope. Among these blessings are the hope of glory (Col. 1:27), the hope of eternal life (Titus 1:2; 3:7), and especially hope in the second coming of Christ itself (1 Thess. 2:19; Titus 2:13; 1 Pet. 1:13). Altogether, the New Testament provides a pervasive and uniform encouragement to Christians to set their hope upon the things of the age to come, which Christ will usher in at his return.

The second aspect of Christian hope that sets it apart from hope in our colloquial speech is that Christian hope is certain and assured. The truth of this is evident from what I just observed about the object of Christian hope. The Christian should not regard the coming of Christ and the resurrection of the body as matters of doubt, but as things sure to take place. Scoffers cast doubt on these events (2 Pet. 3:3–4), but "according to his promise we are waiting for new heavens and a new earth in which righteousness dwells" (2 Pet. 3:13). Our hope is as certain as God's promises are certain. This connection of hope with the promises of God is prominent throughout the New Testament. Paul takes up the theme in Titus 1:2, where he speaks of the "hope of eternal life, which God, who never lies, promised before the ages began." Hebrews 6 speaks in exactly the same way, though at greater length. Since the author desires his readers to have "the full assurance of hope until the end" (Heb. 6:11), he writes that "when God desired to show more convincingly to the heirs of the promise the unchangeable character of his purpose, he guaranteed it with an oath, so that by two unchangeable things, in which it is impossible for God to lie, we who have fled for refuge might have strong encouragement to hold fast to the hope set before us" (Heb. 6:17–18). As if to add all the more to our confidence in the God who never lies, Paul reminds those "who were the first to hope in Christ" (Eph. 1:12) that their inheritance is secure because God has predestined them (Eph. 1:11) and that they "were sealed with the promised Holy Spirit, who is the guarantee of our inheritance until we acquire possession of it . . ." (Eph. 1:13–14). God gives his people reason upon reason to be confident in their hope.

It should be clear by now why faith is the fount of hope. The possible but uncertain hope of colloquial speech requires no faith in God, but Christian hope springs out of the foundation of faith in Christ. Because we trust in Christ unto justification, being declared once and for all righteous before God, we need have no doubt that Christ will richly bless us when he returns. Conversely, without faith and justification we can have no such hope, but only fear of judgment. Perhaps nowhere in Scripture is this relationship between faith and hope more clearly evident than in Romans 4–5. In Romans 4:19–21 Paul speaks of Abraham's faith as rejecting "distrust" and being "fully convinced that God was able to do what he had promised." A verse earlier, however, Paul makes the intriguing statement, "In hope [Abraham] believed against hope, that he should become the father of many nations . . ." (Rom. 4:18). By "against hope" Paul surely means earthly hope: Sarah's having a child at age 90 was not possible in human terms, and hence not a proper object of hope according to our colloquial language. But Abraham had faith in a God who is not confined by earthly, human limitations, and this gave him a hope that defied earthly hope. Paul proceeds to tell us explicitly what Abraham's example means for us: "Therefore, since we have been justified by faith, we have peace with God through our Lord Jesus Christ. Through him we have also obtained access by faith into this grace in which we stand, and we rejoice in hope of the glory of God" (Rom. 5:1–2). Justification by faith, then, produces peace within believers, for they know that they are right with God. In turn, Paul explains, this causes us to rejoice *in hope*, the hope of the glory of God. Several verses later Paul helps us to understand why faith, which receives this blessing of justification *now*, produces hope for the glory of God *in the age to come*: "Since, therefore, we have now been justified by his blood, much more shall we be saved by him from the wrath of God" (Rom. 5:9). Christians have hope because by faith they need not fear God's coming wrath. Thus Paul writes in this context, "hope does not put us to shame" (Rom. 5:5).

Understanding and possessing such a hope promises to shape our perspective on a range of issues in bioethics. Often the challenges of bioethics arise out of the context of suffering, and hence tempt people to despair. Does the future simply look bleak for those burdened by infertility or chronic illness, or is there cause for hope in the midst of these trials? As the world understands it—and all too often Christians think in the same way—there is hope for such people only insofar as medical technology offers remedies for their ailments or if they can adjust their expectations and goals for life in such a way that works around their afflictions. But the Christian hope commended in Scripture is strikingly different. The New Testament writers certainly agree that hope is particularly relevant in times of suffering (e.g., see Rom. 4:18; 5:3–4; 8:20–25; 2 Cor. 1:7; 1 Tim. 5:5; and 1 Pet. 3:15). Christians may rightfully wish that medicine will allow the infertile to conceive and the sick to become healthy, but these are not the objects of their biblical hope. Instead, Christians are to find their hope, in the midst of suffering, in the coming of Christ and the resurrection of their bodies. Medicine may or may not make an ailing body well again temporarily, but the resurrection will, without a doubt, make our bodies whole permanently. Surely this is a far greater kind of hope in time of suffering, but it requires a radical reorientation of the ways in which we tend to think and feel. Our sinful nature tends to be "set on earthly things" (Phil. 3:19), but we ought to live as those whose "citizenship is in heaven" (Phil. 3:20) and whose minds are "on things that are above" (Col. 3:2). Only then can true hope emerge to guide us as we wrestle with the challenges of bioethics.

Love

After considering faith and hope, it is appropriate to turn our attention to the virtue of love. As Paul famously says in 1 Corinthians 13:13, "So now faith, hope, and love abide, these three; but the greatest of these is love." Following all that Paul says about love in the first twelve verses of 1 Corinthians 13, his conclusion about the preeminence of love is not surprising. The order in which Paul lists these virtues also makes sense. Faith is the fount of all the other virtues, hope springs forth from faith, and, as I would argue, love proceeds from faith and hope. Love is the preeminent Christian virtue, not because it can exist independently of faith and hope, but because faith and hope serve as the necessary foundation for love, that supreme work and crowning achievement of the Holy Spirit in the Christian. Faith and hope as we know them now will fade away in the age to come, because we will *see* Christ and our heavenly inheritance, making those virtues unnecessary (see Rom. 8:24–25; 2 Cor. 5:7). But love "never ends" (1 Cor. 13:8). What then is the character of this love, how does it flow from faith and hope, and what does it have to do with bioethics?

As with the concept of "hope," biblical love is rather different from the "love" that we often refer to and hear about in our colloquial speech. Love in colloquial speech frequently refers to a feeling that one person has for another person or thing. If we say that someone loves another person, we generally mean that she has either great fondness for that person (in the case of a friend or family member) or erotic attraction (in the case of a romantic interest). Such love is often thought of as something out of one's own control, as the phrase "falling in love" suggests. Even saying to someone, "I love you," ordinarily gets at the attitude that one feels toward another. Sometimes, of course, a concrete action causes us to talk about love, as when we see a father caring for his sick daughter and speak of him loving her very much. But even then we often take the concrete action not as love itself but as evidence of the feeling of love.

Given this common understanding of love, Scripture's description of love is noteworthy. Certainly Scripture does not deny that love involves a certain feeling or attitude toward another, but its primary focus is on love as action. In Scripture, action is not simply evidence that love is present, but proper action *is* love, or, perhaps better, love *is* right action. Paul says in 1 Corinthians 13:4–5, "Love *is* patient and kind; love does not envy or boast; it is not arrogant or rude. It does not insist on its own way; it is not irritable or resentful." In fact, though Jesus' words in John 14:15 may suggest that love is simply that which stands behind and motivates our other good works ("If you love me, you will keep my commandments"), elsewhere in Scripture we find that love actually *is* the carrying out of all good works. Jesus and Paul both identify love as the sum of the law, and therefore as the content of all our obedience (Matt. 22:36–40; Rom. 13:8–10). Not to murder, not to commit adultery, not to steal, not to bear false witness—that is love. The apostle John, who emphasized the theme of love perhaps more than any other biblical writer, speaks exactly in this way. "For this *is* the love of God, that we keep his commandments . . ." (1 John 5:3), "this *is* love, that we walk according to his commandments . . ." (2 John 6). We love, therefore, precisely by obeying all of God's commands. In this sense, love is not something different from other virtues or obedient acts, but is the bundling of them all into a single package.

Such an understanding of love may threaten to make it a rather unwieldy subject. How can we understand, let alone put into practice, something that is so all-encompassing? Is there any way to define love apart from simply compiling a long list of virtues and obedient actions? I suggest that an accurate and helpful way of defining love is as the giving of *oneself* for the good of another. At the heart of love is self-giving, a self-giving that has many facets that the other virtues and obedient actions express. Theologians sometimes speak about God's love as his goodness expressed in self-giving. Scripture indicates that this is a good way to understand both divine and human love.

This is evident in regard to human love in 1 Corinthians 13:4–5. The characteristics of love—patience and kindness—are other-directed. The descriptions of what love is not—envious, boastful, arrogant, rude— indicate that we should not be so focused upon ourselves. Love, Paul writes, does not "insist on its own way," or, as other translations put it, is not "self-seeking." But surely there is no better illustration of love as self-giving than God's giving his own Son over to death on behalf of sinners, who are not just others, but enemies. In Scripture this expression of divine love is the supreme model for our own love.

Paul reflects on this model in Romans 5:7–8. He begins by reminding us that it is rare to find a person who will give up his life for another, though at times someone will die for a good person. Paul then points us to God, who does what we certainly do not expect: "God shows his love for us in that while we were still sinners, Christ died for us." Shortly thereafter Paul makes this all the more poignant, pointing out that God did this "while we were enemies" (Rom. 5:10). John reasons similarly when he writes, "By this we know love, that he laid down his life for us . . ." (1 John 3:16). But John takes his argument in a direction different from Paul's argument in Romans. John makes clear that God's love should be the model for our own, for he adds immediately thereafter in 1 John 3:16: "and we ought to lay down our lives for the brothers." Later John speaks along the same lines: "In this is love, not that we have loved God but that he loved us and sent his Son to be the propitiation for our sins. Beloved, if God so loved us, we also ought to love one another" (1 John 4:10–11). In light of this we can appreciate the definition of love as self-giving, even as the ultimate self-giving.

At this point we can revisit the idea that Christian love flows from faith (and hope). First John 4:19 says that "we love because he first loved us," indicating that God's love in sending his Son to die is the reason why we must love according to his example. If God's love is the reason for our love, then surely our love must be grounded in faith in this self-giving God. Paul puts this point concisely when he says that the only thing that counts is "faith working through love" (Gal. 5:6). Yet how can this be, especially since non-Christians, without faith in Christ, show great acts of love, even laying down their lives on behalf of others on occasion? Even apart from Scripture, unbelievers know about the kind of love that seeks justice, for God reveals his justice in the natural order and in every human conscience (see Rom. 1:20, 32; 2:14–15). And since God delays the final execution of his justice by preserving this world and bestowing many good things upon it, an expression of love for his enemies (see Matt. 5:44–45), all people can also know something about the kind of love that is tolerant and forbearing, even apart from Scripture. But the fullness of Christian love, which involves true forgiveness of sins and self-giving even unto death, is not something that can be known without biblical revelation. Non-Christians do at times lay down their lives for others—in war, for example—but though we rightly regard such acts as highly admirable, are they not ultimately tragic? What satisfying meaning can be given to such acts if the self-sacrificing person himself has no hope beyond death?

In Christ, however, the Christian finds the highest meaning in self-sacrifice, even when there is no conceivable earthly reward or when death itself is the result. The crucifixion of an unjustly accused Jewish preacher seems to the external eye to be one more senseless act of violence bringing sorrow to yet one more bereaved family. Yet in this event the purpose of history is revealed, as justice and mercy meet in perfect harmony and a lost people is reconciled to God. In this event God makes known that self-sacrifice, so meaningless to earthly eyes, has a blessed resolution. By following the way of mercy, forgiveness, and self-sacrifice that God displayed in Christ, we act in faith that God has justified us, thereby taking away our fear of judgment, and act in hope that God will preserve us beyond the grave unto the resurrection. Through faith and hope, therefore, we know that forgiveness and self-sacrifice need not mean defeat, but through the blessing of God's benevolent providence bring about much good, even the triumph of God's plans in history. Through faith and hope we know that our treasure is in heaven, which reminds us that we must not cling selfishly to the things of this world.

What does this Christian vision of love have to do with bioethics? At a very general level, possessing the virtue of love helps to preserve us against the strong temptation in many situations to be obsessed about our own condition. Our own infertility, our own illness, or our own looming death often threatens to make us impervious to others, so overwhelming do our own problems seem. Yet not only must we think of others in the midst of our own suffering, but we must also take account of how the decisions we make while we suffer often deeply affect others. In subsequent chapters I discuss the degree to which decisions about things such as having children and accepting or refusing treatment are decisions that we should make in the context of our various communities and not as solitary individuals. We might also think of bioethical emergencies. If we are called upon to make a quick decision about how to treat (or not to treat) a comatose loved one, we may immediately ask ourselves what is the compassionate thing to do. But when there is no time for reflection or for consulting a trusted advisor, it is critical that we be the right sort of person, with the right virtues. Surely a person who has long been cultivating the virtue of love will know, much better than one who has not, what compassion demands in such a difficult situation.

Courage

Faith, hope, and love, in some sense, provide a comprehensive picture of the Christian virtues. Faith is the fount, hope is its fruit, and love, which encompasses all other virtues, flows from them. But while all other virtues are indeed the expression of love, certain virtues seem especially important in the context of bioethics, and thus deserve their own consideration. Two of these are courage and contentment. We will consider what courage and contentment are, how they are rooted in faith and hope, and, at an initial level, what they have to do with bioethics. I will then discuss wisdom, which deserves a separate treatment.

What is courage? Courage is often understood as the virtue of pursuing what is good in the face of danger and hardship, and this definition is consistent with the kind of courage commended in Scripture. Several matters relating to this definition need clarification, however, for secular and other religious conceptions of courage are by no means identical to Christian courage.

One matter in need of clarification is the relation of courage to fear. Many writers define courage as facing danger or hardship *without fear*, or even as a synonym for *fearlessness*. I purposely left fear out of my definition of courage, because I do not believe that most people think of courage as involving the absence of fear. On the contrary, to exhibit courage, as commonly understood, a person must have a certain kind of fear, a fear that displays a proper sense of what is truly dangerous. We might imagine a soldier on the front lines who rushes into battle with bullets flying around him with no sense that his life may end at any moment. Such a man would be judged reckless and naïve, but surely not courageous. Or we might imagine the same soldier perfectly aware that death may be imminent but somehow feeling no fear of dying. In such a case, rushing into battle is really no different for him from eating a sandwich—neither provokes any sense of fear. It is difficult to see how, for this man, rushing into battle is any more courageous than eating that sandwich. Certainly courage involves an ability to control and moderate one's fears, but without any fear there is no need for courage in the first place.

Another point of clarification is that courage requires a proper sense of what good things are worth pursuing at the cost of danger and hardship. We ordinarily associate courage with the person who tells the truth even when she knows that her career will suffer or with the person who rushes into battle for the sake of defending his country. Most people acknowledge truth and national defense as goods worth suffering for. But what if we imagine the person who attempts to jump his bicycle over a wide, gaping canyon in order to impress his girlfriend? Since there is no good being pursued that is in any sense proportional to the risk undertaken, we would judge this person to be reckless and foolhardy, not courageous.

A final point left unclear in the definition of courage concerns its source. In other words, where does a person get courage in order to endure fearful things for the sake of pursuing what is good and right? Here the common consensus about courage breaks down. The classic Stoic answer was that courage comes from detachment, making oneself indifferent toward the things of the outside world. Gaining such detachment might in fact be effective in emboldening someone to tell the truth at the cost of her job, for this detachment presumably makes her employment situation a matter of little concern. But a Christian conception of courage is quite different. While Stoic courage presumes that the world outside of oneself is unimportant, Christian courage acknowledges other people and indeed the world as a whole to be very important. This raises the question of what is distinctive about the courage commanded in Scripture and brings us back again to the foundational character of faith and hope.

What is distinctive about the Christian view of courage is that the will of God determines what is good and worth pursuing, and our faith in the promises of God and our hope rooted in the eschatological future give us the courage to persevere in this pursuit. In the Old Testament some of the most memorable exhortations to courage come as the Israelites are about to enter the Promised Land. Entering Canaan clearly evoked fear in their hearts, for forty years earlier fear of the native inhabitants had overcome their fathers, and they disobeyed the Lord by refusing to go in (Num. 13:25–14:10; Deut. 1:19–33). In the face of this fear, God called upon the new generation to have courage and thus to do everything that he had commanded them: "Be strong and courageous, for you shall cause this people to inherit the land that I swore to their fathers to give them. Only be strong and very courageous, being careful to do according to all the law that Moses my servant commanded. . . . Be strong and courageous. Do not be frightened, and do not be dismayed, for the LORD your God is with you wherever you go" (Josh. 1:6–7, 9). The good worth pursuing was God's law, and the source of this boldness was the fact that God had sworn to prosper them if they obeyed him.

This Old Testament call to courage, therefore, involved a context that we still often associate with courage—going to battle—and rested upon the distinctive promises made to Israel, promises that guaranteed success and prosperity in the Promised Land if they obeyed. But throughout the Old Testament Israel constantly disobeyed, and their courage failed. In light of this background, Paul rejoices that God has made a new and better covenant with his people in these last days, a covenant that will bring lasting glory (2 Cor. 3:7–11), and he therefore concludes: "Since we have such a *hope*, we are very bold" (2 Cor. 3:12). In Christ, all of God's promises are "Yes" (2 Cor. 1:20), and our eyes are set not on an earthly land to be enjoyed because of our own obedience but on a heavenly, eschatological kingdom to be enjoyed because of Christ's obedience once and for all. Later in 2 Corinthians Paul reflects on the heavenly dwelling that we have beyond death, the swallowing up of mortality by life, and the Holy Spirit's presence with us as a guarantee (2 Cor. 5:1–5), all of which cause him to say: "So we are always of good courage" (2 Cor. 5:6). What gave Paul this courage, even though he did not yet see or possess this eternal life? He called upon his *faith*: "We walk by faith, not by sight" (2 Cor. 5:7). Bolstered by this faith in Christ and looking ahead to his eschatological hope, Paul was courageous in undertaking the work set before him: "Yes, we are of good courage, and we would rather be away from the body and at home with the Lord. So whether we are at home or away, we make it our aim to please him" (2 Cor. 5:8–9). Elsewhere Paul similarly expresses courage in the face of death, rooted in the hope of his everlasting welfare, which gives him strength to press on in the work entrusted to him (see Phil. 1:20–24). Paul's reasoning in Philippians 1, in fact, helps us to understand how courage, rooted in faith and hope, is itself an act of love. It is an act of love not only toward God, whose will we follow even amidst the threat of great loss, but in many cases also toward our neighbor, whose welfare we must seek even when it may hinder our own welfare. Paul points to an excellent example of such loving courage in action when he holds Epaphroditus in the highest esteem for risking his life both for the sake of Christ and for the sake of Paul's relationship with the Philippian church (Phil. 2:29–30).

In short, Scripture recognizes that there are things that we understandably fear, especially death. As we considered in chapter 2, God does not promise to relieve us of dangers, hardships, and sufferings in this life. But he has justified us by faith and has given us the hope of life everlasting, promising to be with us forever and to work out all things for our good. Resting in his promises and knowing especially that the last and greatest enemy, death, has been defeated, we have courage to face these things that we fear. Christians must seek their courage not from their own personal resources or from a sense of detachment from the world, as the Stoic would have it, but from the objective, concrete promises of God that sustain us through objective, concrete dangers.

We will later consider the importance of courage for bioethics. For now I note that bioethical decisions ordinarily arise in the context of suffering and loss, that is, in the face of things that we fear. Scripture does not sustain us through these things by telling us that our suffering is not real or that our fear is illegitimate. Indeed, it treats things such as illness and especially death as evils that are naturally fearful. As we anticipate momentous decisions about whether or how we treat an illness or about how we die, we must cultivate Christian courage so that these decisions are not driven by fear of evil but by a desire to do what is right, a desire that can withstand the temptation to be diverted from the proper course by inordinate desire to avoid what we fear.

Contentment

Contentment is the virtue by which we submit to and find peace in God's will for our condition in every circumstance of life. This is a distinctively Christian definition, but it is worth reflecting for a moment on what the idea of contentment communicates in our ordinary language. Contentment in fact is not even universally recognized as a virtue. People sometimes regard contentment as simply a natural disposition that some individuals have and some do not. In this sense, a contented person might be contrasted with an ambitious person, and in many cases the ambitious person is more widely admired than the contented one (who might be regarded as unmotivated or lazy). Another significant suspicion cast upon contentment comes from those concerned about the dispossessed and marginalized in society. Is recommending contentment to those who are deprived of basic rights and opportunities a way of keeping them down and maintaining the advantages of the privileged? Along these lines, contentment should be discouraged, and people should be encouraged to overcome barriers.

Defining contentment as finding peace in God's will in every circumstance and interpreting this in the light of Christian faith, hope, and love, should help us to appreciate contentment in a proper sense, as a virtue and not as a natural disposition or tool of the privileged. Scripture most readily associates contentment with times of earthly deprivation, as Paul's exhortations often demonstrate (see 2 Cor. 8:2; 9:8; Phil. 4:11–12; 1 Tim. 6:6–8). But we should not forget that discontentment can manifest itself in every experience of life. The vices that stand most clearly opposed to contentment, such as grumbling, envy, and covetousness, afflict all sorts of people, whether healthy or sick, rich or poor. Discontentment may offer special temptations in time of serious need, but inordinate desire for more than we have is a sin against which all must guard.

Whatever the earthly condition in which we find ourselves, the biblical remedy for discontentment is not the promise that we will get what we want. In other words, Scripture does not instruct Christians to be content in illness because they will recover, to be content in poverty because they will become rich, or to be content in a bad marriage because the relationship with one's spouse will soon heal. Scripture presents the Christian's life in this age as one of suffering, as a pilgrimage away from our everlasting home, and consequently there is no guarantee that any particular hardship that we experience will go away this side of the resurrection. I hasten to add, in part as a response to the critics of contentment mentioned above, that having contentment does not prevent us from pursuing remedies for earthly hardships. Christians certainly may (and many times *should*) use morally permissible means to alleviate illness, poverty, and troubled marriage relationships. But what makes contentment—at least *Christian* contentment—such a wonderful yet challenging thing is that it exists alongside of our legitimate attempts to improve our earthly condition. In other words, contentment involves finding peace in our hardships even while we strive to eliminate them. Contentment is compatible with attempts to alleviate suffering, but its power lies in submitting to and finding peace in God's will whether or not the immediate alleviation of suffering is part of that will.

As with the other virtues, the source and foundation of contentment is faith and hope. Christian contentment springs only from this soil. Only the person with faith in the God who justifies and with hope in the resurrection at Christ's second coming can know true contentment. Perhaps nowhere is this so evident as in Paul's remarkable statement about his own contentment in Philippians 4:11–12. He writes: "Not that I am speaking of being in need, for I have learned in whatever situation I am to be content. I know how to be brought low, and I know how to abound. In any and every circumstance, I have learned the secret of facing plenty and hunger, abundance and need." Simply read by themselves, these words seem too good to be true, too confident to be credible. Such Christian contentment *is* remarkable and even incredible from an earthly perspective. These words of Paul do not float in a vacuum, however, but follow a memorable description of where his faith and hope lie. In Philippians 3:1–9 Paul recounts a time when he put confidence in himself and in his own achievements. But now he considers all of these achievements a loss and rubbish "in order that I may gain Christ and be found in him, not having a righteousness of my own that comes from the law, but that which comes through *faith* in Christ, the righteousness from God that depends on *faith*" (Phil. 3:8–9). In other words, Paul has found confidence in the justification that he has already obtained, through faith and based on Christ's own righteousness. Having established that, Paul turns immediately to his hope, to that which he has not yet obtained (see Phil. 3:12), that is, his own resurrection that shares in the power of Christ's resurrection: "that I may know him and the power of his resurrection, and may share his sufferings, becoming like him in his death, that by any means possible I may attain the resurrection from the dead" (Phil. 3:10–11). In the following passages he continues to reflect upon the imminent coming of Christ and its bearing upon the way he lives now (see Phil. 3:13–14, 20–21; 4:5). Hence Paul's statement that he has learned to be content in every circumstance is comprehensible. His contentment does not rest in the material things he possessed or would possess in this life, but in what is unseen: his present justification by faith and the hope of his resurrection, with abundant material blessings, at Christ's coming. Such blessings are *staggeringly great*. What Christian, contemplating these things, should not say: "The lines have fallen for me in pleasant places; indeed, I have a beautiful inheritance" (Ps. 16:6)?

   This attitude, of course, is easier described than lived, and the need for contentment should never be invoked to minimize the reality of suffering. But the same person who pointed us to the unseen things of faith and hope as the source of contentment suffered terrible things himself (see 2 Cor. 11:24–29), and he certainly did not speak out of ignorance or naiveté. Paul was no Stoic. He even pleaded with the Lord to relieve him of one particular burden, to which the Lord responded, "My grace is sufficient for you . . ." (2 Cor. 12:8–9). He had to endure this burden, yet he concluded: "For the sake of Christ, then, I am content with weaknesses, insults, hardships, persecutions, and calamities. For when I am weak, then I am strong" (2 Cor. 12:10). Paul recognized that his own weakness was God's tool for glorifying himself and advancing the gospel, and in this he was content.

Paul's reflections in 2 Corinthians 11–12 concern his role as an apostle of Christ, a role that no one today is called to serve. But the general point that our times of suffering serve God's beneficent purposes is still of great relevance for growing in the virtue of contentment. God's ways are often mysterious, leaving us unable to understand fully his purposes in the things that we experience. Yet we know that God sanctifies us (that is, mortifies sin and brings forth holiness within us) through our sufferings, as we endure them in faith and hope (see Rom. 5:1–5; James 1:2–8). We rightly desire sanctification and pray to God that he would sanctify us—and thus we should strive to be content when he satisfies such desires and answers such prayers in ways that we would not choose. Paul reminds us that we will indeed receive the grace of God as we exhibit contentment in times of want: "God is able to make all grace abound to you, so that having all sufficiency [the original Greek word here means *contentment*] in all things at all times, you may abound in every good work" (2 Cor. 9:8). This abundance of grace is not in the service of satisfying whatever our earthly desires might be, but for enabling us to do good works and to meet the needs *of others*, which in turn evokes praise and thanksgiving *toward God* (2 Cor. 9:8–15). Our contentment, then, for the sake of others' good and God's praise, is truly an act of love, toward both God and our neighbor. If we trust God's promise that he will sanctify us, build his church, and bring glory to himself, then we should also trust that the way in which he does so is wise and gracious, and find contentment *in him* however that way leads.

The virtue of contentment is crucial for bioethics in large part because bioethical questions usually emerge as a result of dissatisfaction with our current state of affairs. Bioethics concerns things that we desire but lack (such as children or health) and concerns the difficult moral questions that arise from possible solutions. Given our discussion, the Christian's first responsibility in such circumstances is to learn contentment in whatever condition she experiences (such as infertility or illness), accepting that God may not will to relieve her from it. Then, from this perspective of contentment, the Christian should consider morally permissible ways to remedy her condition. I would argue, moreover, that true contentment may significantly alter our perspective on the dilemmas we face and it may even persuade us, at times, that remaining in our undesired condition is the most ethically satisfying decision.

Wisdom

Wisdom is a virtue of profound importance for bioethics. To this point I have attempted to show the connection among various virtues, portraying faith as the fount of all the others. Wisdom breaks this pattern in some sense. Scripture recognizes that genuine wisdom existed among peoples in the ancient world who did not worship the true God (see 1 Kings 4:30; Acts 7:22). Confirming this truth, recent scholarship has discovered significant similarities between the biblical wisdom literature (such as Proverbs) and the wisdom literature of Israel's pagan neighbors. The quest for wisdom and the discovery of wisdom, therefore, were not unique to Old Testament Israel. Old Testament wisdom literature, furthermore, though given to Israel as the covenant community, sets forth the way of wisdom largely without explicit reference to the reality of redemption. That is to say, Scripture explains the way of wisdom to some degree independently of God's saving grace. At the same time, the New Testament also tells us that the Lord Jesus Christ is *the* Wisdom of God (1 Cor. 1:24) and points to *the cross of Christ* as the supreme demonstration of God's wisdom, a wisdom that is foolishness in the eyes of the world (1 Cor. 1:18–2:15). Christians "have the mind of Christ" (1 Cor. 2:16). Faith in Christ, therefore, is obviously crucial to becoming a person of wisdom in the fullest sense. Genuine wisdom is possible without saving faith in the true God, but the deepest, most profound wisdom comes only in Christ. God's work in Christ displays a wisdom that the observation of nature and human ingenuity could never discover: a way of saving sinners that displays God's mercy and justice simultaneously.

What then is wisdom and why is it necessary? Perhaps a helpful general definition is that wisdom is the ability to understand how the world works. Occasionally in Scripture wisdom refers to a broad understanding that extends to matters of natural science (see 1 Kings 4:33), but ordinarily wisdom is a matter of *moral* knowledge and practice. Proverbs commends a wisdom that understands human nature, human conduct, and human relationships. It perceives the relationship between certain kinds of actions and certain kinds of consequences. Wisdom apprehends a broader moral order in the world, and it determines how particular ethical decisions fit (or do not fit) into that order. Such wisdom is not an alternative to knowledge of moral rules or to the cultivation of virtues, but virtues and knowledge of rules are not able to function on their own, without wisdom. Rules can never be exhaustive, anticipating every possible moral situation. Virtues are meant to be exercised in a complex and often puzzling world. Wisdom enables a person to put her virtues into concrete practice and to apply her moral rules in real life. Wisdom provides the ability to perceive how one's virtues and principles can come to proper expression in particular circumstances.

Thus wisdom is necessary for at least two general reasons. First, knowing moral rules is necessary but insufficient for making proper ethical decisions in the concrete circumstances of life. Even Scripture's rules are not so exhaustive that they leave no need to apply them to specific situations. It is wisdom that guides us in applying them. Second, we often know *what* moral goals we are trying to attain but do not know *how* to attain them. Wisdom helps us to understand what sort of conduct conduces to reaching our moral goals. For example, the book of Proverbs speaks extensively about what sort of behavior promotes peace among neighbors, sexual chastity, and financial prosperity. We do not necessarily need wisdom to know that these are good things to attain, but we do need wisdom to understand how to attain them as we navigate the maze of life. Wisdom achieves this by enabling us to perceive the world in its interrelating parts and thereby to anticipate the kinds of consequences that tend to flow from particular actions.

How is such wisdom attained? Scripture points us to two things that we might call religious requirements for attaining wisdom: the fear of the Lord and prayer. Scripture speaks of the fear of the Lord as foundational for wisdom, perhaps most famously in Proverbs 1:7 and Job 28:28. One of the reasons for this is that the fear of God ought to instill a corresponding humility, and "with the humble is wisdom" (Prov. 11:2). A person who is self-absorbed and able only to see things from the perspective of his own interests will never be able to understand other people and thus how the broader moral order fits together, the very things that wisdom involves. The fear of God and its corresponding humility, therefore, are crucial for obtaining wisdom. Prayer is also necessary for the attainment of wisdom, as James 1:5 counsels: "If any of you lacks wisdom, let him ask God, who gives generously to all without reproach, and it will be given him."

Though Scripture points us to the fear of God and prayer as foundational for obtaining wisdom, we do injustice to the larger biblical witness if we leave matters there. Proverbs makes clear that people obtain wisdom only as they make their way thoughtfully and reflectively through the various experiences of life. Wisdom does not drop suddenly from heaven apart from going through life, learning from it, and learning from those who have experienced it before us. Proverbs repeatedly tells us, for example, that we should listen to our parents and elders, that we should seek out advice before making decisions (from multiple counselors), and that we should observe and learn from the behavior of animals, and it points to many other practical ways to gain insight into the way things work. Only when we live such humble, thoughtful, and reflective lives can we expect God to bless our prayers for wisdom.

Wisdom is relevant for every part of our lives, but it has a special relevance in bioethical decision making. In few areas of contemporary life is it more obvious than in bioethics that Scripture does not provide a specific answer to every moral problem. In the past two chapters we have been exploring many things that Scripture teaches that are relevant to bioethics, but about in vitro fertilization, cloning, stem cells, ventilators, and feeding tubes Scripture says not a word. The doctrines, rules, and virtues commended in Scripture must be applied to circumstances unknown to the biblical writers, and without a great measure of wisdom bioethics will remain a murky endeavor. In addition, bioethical decisions require a great deal of attention to particular circumstances. Biblical wisdom trains us to observe details, recognizing that a small change in circumstance may require a significant change in response. To make morally sound bioethical decisions we must understand the precise nature of the problem, the available remedies, and the likely consequences of those remedies. Since most people have limited medical and scientific knowledge, they must depend upon physicians and other experts in order to obtain such information. We must seek out advice, weigh different opinions, and anticipate the consequences of our decisions—the very things that wisdom entails. Whether they are wrestling with bioethics at the beginning or at the end of life, Christians must be wise if they are to make responsible moral decisions.

Conclusion

We have explored several of the Christian virtues necessary for sound bioethical decision making. Scripture calls us not only to act in certain ways but also to *be* a certain kind of people. If we are to put into practice the kind of life that Scripture commends, then we must be the kind of people who are able to do so. The whole Christian life demands development in the virtues, and those who are growing in the virtues are equipped to respond to difficult bioethical decisions in ways that the nonvirtuous are not. As we address particular bioethical problems at the beginning and end of life, we will return often to reflect upon how these virtues should shape our responses to the challenges of contemporary bioethics.

PART 2

THE BEGINNING OF LIFE

Some of the most controversial bioethics debates concern the purpose of marriage, procreation and assisted reproduction, and the nature and status of human life in its earliest days. These matters touch upon decisions that a great many Christians will face personally at some point in their lives—especially decisions related to conceiving and bearing children—and many of them have become controversial political topics in recent years, such as cloning, stem-cell research, and especially abortion. It is tempting for writers who deal with these issues to focus on rather abstract questions. Are there good philosophical arguments for affirming that a human embryo is a person with a right to life? Does use of artificial contraception violate the inherent meaning of sex? While it is helpful and even necessary to address questions like these when investigating matters of abortion and contraception, I seek to place the matters before us in the context of the broader Christian life. Decisions about limiting the number of their children, pursuing medical help in the face of infertility, and protecting their unborn children are all choices that confront Christians in the midst of their ongoing Christian lives and that can never be viewed apart from them.

The three chapters in Part 2 explore a variety of beginning-of-life issues in the context of Christian faith and life. Chapter 4 begins with a discussion of marriage and of remaining unmarried that will be foundational to all three chapters. This chapter proceeds to reflect upon the human task of procreation and upon Christians' choices and obligations in the face of the wide variety of contraceptive options available today that invite them to limit proactively the size of their families. Chapter 5 turns to one of the most trying circumstances that a married couple can confront: infertility. This chapter discusses the proper attitude toward infertility and assisted reproduction that arises from a well-lived Christian life and then investigates the propriety of some specific assisted-reproduction options. Finally, chapter 6 explores the socially divisive question about the status of the human embryo. Although, in keeping with the plan of this book, I will not offer judgments or strategies regarding public policy per se, I do consider what view of the embryo is consistent with Christian faith and life, a view that must shape Christians' personal decisions and that will surely influence their participation in public affairs.

4

MARRIAGE, PROCREATION, AND CONTRACEPTION

Historically Christians have understood all things related to sex, procreation, and bearing children in relation to marriage. A consideration of marriage is therefore essential background for examining matters such as contraception, assisted reproduction, and treatment of the embryo in the broader context of the Christian life.

The Nature and Purpose of Marriage

Christians have affirmed that sexual intimacy is the exclusive domain of the marriage relationship and have cast a wary eye at technological developments that separate sexual intimacy from the procreation of children. Recent cultural trends in the West include significant increases in the divorce rate, the widespread acceptance of sexual relationships outside of the marriage bond, and even fundamental shifts in the understanding of who may marry whom (I write this in California the day after the state began issuing marriage licenses to homosexual couples). A theologically sound perspective on marriage can no longer be assumed in the broader culture, nor even among many professing Christians and churches, which often manifest the same trends as the world around them in regard to family breakdown and sexual impropriety. We therefore need to consider some basic theological truths about the marriage relationship and some important matters concerning the state of *not* being married.

The Purposes and Meaning of Marriage

Scripture identifies four distinct but related purposes of marriage. The Westminster Confession of Faith helpfully summarizes them: "for the mutual help of husband and wife, for the increase of mankind with legitimate issue, and of the church with an holy seed; and for the preventing of uncleanness" (WCF 24.2). The first of these purposes, the mutual help of husband and wife, is evident in Genesis 2:18–24, where God observes that it is not good for Adam to be alone and thus creates Eve as "a helper fit for him." Scripture speaks of the second purpose, the increase of mankind, in Genesis 1:27–28. After referring to his image bearers as "male and female," God commands them to "be fruitful and multiply." This task of procreating and populating the earth is a task *common* to the human race. God ordained marriage and procreation at the beginning and reaffirmed this mandate in his covenant with Noah (Gen. 9:1, 7). This Noahic covenant was made not with believers only but with *all* of Noah's descendents, and even "every living creature" (9:9–10, 15–16). Marriage and childbearing are common to believers and unbelievers alike, and thus the marriage of two unbelievers is no less valid in the sight of God than that of two believers. One reason that God ordained marriage was to provide a context for raising children and thus populating the whole earth.

The third purpose of marriage, the provision of the church with a holy seed, is obviously related to the previous purpose but also distinct from it. Though believers and unbelievers share the common, God-ordained task of multiplying and filling the earth, believers have the additional privilege of bearing children who are members of the church and thus contribute to its ongoing growth and prosperity. Already from the days of Abraham God reckoned the children of believers as members of the redemptive covenant community (Gen. 17:7–14), and the New Testament as well considers children members of the church (e.g., Matt. 19:13–15; Eph. 6:1–3). While the church does not create the marriage relationship, it recognizes the good and God-ordained character of marriage and welcomes the children of believing parents. As the prophet Malachi wrote, "Did he not make them one, with a portion of the Spirit in their union? And what was the one God seeking? Godly offspring. So guard yourselves in your spirit, and let none of you be faithless to the wife of your youth" (Mal. 2:15).

Finally, Scripture presents marriage as designed by God to "prevent uncleanness." This reflects the fact that we are sexual creatures who seek to express our sexuality for its own sake and not only for the purpose of procreating. The language "prevent uncleanness" alludes to Paul's admonition to spouses not to refrain from regular sexual relations, "because of the temptation to sexual immorality" (1 Cor. 7:1–9). Regular marital relations lessen the temptation to engage in nonmarital sexual activity. But this purpose of marriage should not be viewed negatively, as if sexual relations are inherently evil and marriage simply keeps a person from falling into greater sin. God created human beings as sexual creatures, and it is a *good* thing to express this aspect of our nature in the proper way, that is, in the context of a life-long, exclusive commitment between a man and woman. The Song of Solomon provides ample illustration of the goodness and delight that a wholesome sexual relationship brings.

In chapter 2 we explored biblical teaching on the image of God. This teaching is highly relevant when considering marriage, for the marriage relationship permits spouses to reflect the image of God in unique ways. To bear God's image is to be a social creature. There are many ways outside of marriage to engage in social relations, of course, but the marriage of a man and woman was the original human social relationship (Gen. 1:27). Our first and primary relationship is with God, not with other human beings, and the marital relationship reflects this basic divine-human relationship more profoundly than any other intrahuman relationship does. As each person's relationship with God is to be perpetual, intimate, and exclusive (for we are to have *no* other gods beside him), so the husband-wife relationship is to be perpetual (until death), intimate (including sexually), and exclusive (hence the prohibition of adultery). Relationships among friends or among parents and children are immensely meaningful, but they need not be perpetual (in the case of friends) or exclusive (since one may have more than one friend, child, or parent), and must not be sexually intimate. The marriage relationship also expresses the image in a unique way in that it ordinarily entails pro*creation*. The first twenty-five verses of Genesis 1 highlight the fruitfulness of God the Creator, as he brings all things into being out of nothing. Then, when he creates men and women in his image, he commands them to be fruitful and multiply. Like their God, image bearers are to be fruitful, and though they cannot create things out of nothing, the emergence of a child through the union of a man and woman comes as close to this as anything we can imagine.

Christianity and Remaining Unmarried

According to Scripture, therefore, marriage is an exalted state. But it is not the only God-pleasing state in which we can live. While the church does well to affirm marriage and childbearing, it often does a disservice to many of its members by marginalizing the nonmarried and the childless. This can happen in various ways. For example, it can happen when churches advertise themselves as being *family* friendly or as supporting *family* values, even when many of their members do not have a family, at least not a spouse or children. It can happen when churches treat unmarried adults simply as those who are not *yet* married, as if their lives are in a holding pattern until marriage brings meaning to them. It can happen when Christians segregate their social lives, as if people who are married with children should primarily associate with each other and unmarried people with each other (and, when they do mingle, by people talking incessantly about their children as if those without children find such conversations just as fascinating as they do). It can happen when Christians raise girls as if being a wife and mother is the only worthy goal to pursue in life, such that those who do not marry and have children feel that they have somehow failed and are unprepared to find other valuable things to do.

My comments concerning marriage and the image of God may seem to perpetuate such a disservice to the unmarried and childless, since I argue that the marital relationship offers opportunity to reflect the image of God in unique ways. The image of God, however, is a complex reality, as discussed in chapter 2. Human beings were created for the task of exercising dominion over creation (Gen. 1:26), yet no human being can participate in every aspect of this task. The unmarried and childless often have opportunities to engage in various culture pursuits that, for one reason or another, those who have responsibilities of spouse and children do not have. No one individual can express the image of God comprehensively, and in this sense the unmarried are no different from the married. When we consider that the Lord Jesus Christ, *the* image of the Father (Col. 1:15; Heb. 1:3), remained unmarried and without children throughout his earthly life, we should not be quick to relegate the unmarried and childless to anything resembling an inferior position.

This conclusion is confirmed by the New Testament's praise of the nonmarried state and its lack of a single reference to barrenness as a tragedy or curse (the only exception being Luke 1:7, which I will discuss later). This stands in remarkable contrast to the Old Testament, which says nothing favorable about being unmarried and which presents barrenness as a terrible affliction. Profound theological reasons underlie this shift from Old to New Testament, and we do well to avoid clinging to an Old Testament perspective that misses how the coming of Jesus Christ has liberated his people from the curse of barrenness.

Immediately after the fall of Adam and Eve, God promised that deliverance would come through the "offspring" of the woman, who would crush the head of the serpent's offspring (Gen. 3:15). Childbearing was therefore linked to the advent of salvation. The hope of a promised seed shaped the meaning of barrenness in Sarah's famous struggle with childlessness. The failure to bear a child meant the failure of God's redemptive promise to raise up a deliverer and to make Abraham's descendants as numerous as the stars in the sky (Gen. 15:1–6; Gal. 3:16). Furthermore, when God brought Israel into the Promised Land, he allotted an inheritance to each tribe and family (Joshua 13–19). Special rules regulated the way in which Israelites could handle their property in the land. They were not permitted to sell it outside of their families and tribes (see Lev. 25:8–17; Num. 36:7–9; 1 Kings 21:1–3), and they handled with great urgency situations in which a family's possession of a plot of ground was in danger due to the family dying out (see Numbers 36).

The short explanation for this is that the Promised Land was a pledge of something much greater to come, a heavenly Promised Land (Heb. 11:8–16). It was by enjoying the bounty of Canaan, with each sitting under his own vine and fig tree, that the Old Testament saints enjoyed communion with the greater, heavenly realities that they would one day enjoy. For Israelites in the Promised Land, therefore, being childless robbed them of the opportunity to participate in the fulfillment of the Abrahamic promises in two ways. It prevented them from contributing offspring to Abraham's multitude of descendants, and it threatened to cut off a family line from its inheritance,

the divine pledge of eternal life. For this reason it is no wonder that
the Old Testament never presents nonmarriage as a viable option,
considers barrenness a profound curse, and proclaims in the Psalms:
"Behold, children are a heritage from the LORD, the fruit of the womb
a reward. Like arrows in the hand of a warrior are the children of
one's youth. Blessed is the man who fills his quiver with them! . . ."
(Ps. 127:3–5).

Against this background we can appreciate why so many Old Testament stories of God's ongoing work of salvation involve a barren woman giving birth to a child: Isaac, Jacob, Joseph, Samson, and
Samuel. In part this reminded God's people that he had promised to
save them once and for all through the "offspring of the woman," the
"seed of Abraham." It also reminded them that salvation is *God's* work,
not a human work. God performs what human ingenuity could not:
he makes a barren woman give birth. This storyline continued into
the beginning of the New Testament with the conception and birth
of John the Baptist, the last of the Old Testament prophets (Luke
1:5–25; Matt. 11:7–15). Then it came to its climax in a conception
more astounding than that of a barren woman. Indeed, the *virgin* Mary
was the ultimate barren woman, the one whose conception was the
most humanly inexplicable. In this climactic birth God fulfilled once
and for all his promises to Adam and to Abraham, and through them
to all of his people. He brought forth a Son, not by human power but
by divine power, and this Son would indeed "save his people from
their sins" (Matt. 1:21).

Now that God's own Son has been born and has accomplished his
saving work, God's people should never again look at barrenness in the
same way. Galatians 4:4–7 teaches that because of the Son's coming,
we have been adopted by God so that we are now heirs—no longer
heirs of an earthly plot of ground but of the heavenly kingdom itself.
Family and family relations of course remain very important for Christians in the New Testament, but their importance is relativized. When
his mother and brothers came to see him, Jesus looked at those sitting
around him and stated: "Here are my mother and my brothers! For
whoever does the will of God, he is my brother and sister and mother"
(Mark 3:34–35). Our entrance into the church through Christ's work
has incorporated us into a new family, the very "household" of God
(Eph. 2:19; 1 Tim. 3:15). Our new family has higher priority than our
natural families, and if the choice must be made, we ought to forsake

our natural families for the sake of Christ and his church (see Matt. 10:35–37). When the prophet contemplated the coming salvation of God he could even proclaim: "Sing, O barren one, who did not bear; break forth into singing and cry aloud, you who have not been in labor! For the children of the desolate one will be more than the children of her who is married . . ." (Isa. 54:1). Shortly thereafter Isaiah adds: "For thus says the LORD: 'To the eunuchs who keep my Sabbaths, who choose the things that please me and hold fast my covenant, I will give in my house and within my walls a monument and a name better than sons and daughters; I will give them an everlasting name that shall not be cut off'" (Isa. 56:4–5).

Thus Christians, while promoting the good of marriage and "family values," should of all people be the most eager to uphold the good of *not* marrying and having children, even if most Christians do not follow this route. On several occasions in 1 Corinthians 7 Paul states that remaining unmarried can be a better option for believers (1 Cor. 7:1, 7–8, 26, 40), because the present age is passing away (1 Cor. 7:26–31) and because of the desire for undivided devotion to the Lord (1 Cor. 7:32–35). The marginalization of the unmarried and childless, whether direct or subtle, should surely have no place in the church. A proper perspective on these things, furthermore, helps to shape our view on procreation, contraception, and especially assisted reproduction.

Preliminary Reflections on Procreation

Many writers have documented the striking shift in Western society's views of sex and procreation in recent generations. From time immemorial people have sought ways to prevent pregnancy without giving up sex, but with the advent of effective contraceptives, and especially oral contraceptives, otherwise fertile people can now engage in regular sexual activity with a reasonable certainty that pregnancy will not result. Even more recently, the development of artificial means of reproduction, such as artificial insemination and in vitro fertilization, has offered to infertile people the prospect of having children apart from ordinary sexual intercourse. What are often described as the "unitive" and "procreative" aspects of a marital relationship have been separated in ways never before imagined. People have always known that sex does not *always* produce children, but now sex *need not* produce children. Sex always used to be required to produce children, but now children may be conceived apart from sexual relations. Many find this liberating. Others find it disturbing. In light of their broader Christian commitments, how ought believers to evaluate this new situation in which sex and procreation are increasingly separated?

There has been no uniform Christian answer, and this is not surprising, because important theological truths seem to pull us in different directions. On the one hand, Christians confess that the natural connection between sex and procreation is God's design, not the product of an impersonal evolutionary process. God created man male and female (Gen. 1:27), to be united in a relationship of "one flesh" (Gen. 2:24), with the obligation to be "fruitful and multiply" (Gen. 1:28). God intentionally and purposefully sustained this aspect of human nature after the fall into sin, even though it must bear the effects of the curse (Gen. 3:16; 9:1, 7). On the other hand, God also created us to exercise dominion over the earth (Gen. 1:28), and again God sustained, in fallen form, the ability of human beings to develop the potentialities within nature and to produce technological achievements (e.g., Gen. 4:20–22). God created human beings not simply to live *au naturel*, therefore, but to work creatively upon nature and, in some sense, to transcend its limitations. Human beings use their image-bearing capacities to manipulate all sorts of natural events. Is our present technological ability to separate sex and procreation simply an amazing expression of our God-given capacities or a transgression of the way in which God intended human beings to act?

We must reflect on the answers to such questions, and these answers must be properly nuanced. Scripture does not provide any direct instruction about contraception or reproductive technology. This puts a high premium on the exercise of wisdom and discretion for Christians reflecting on what is at stake in particular circumstances. The separation of sex and procreation cannot be condemned simply because it is "unnatural," but we should not think that there is nothing to lose if we go down this road. The shift in perspective from pro*creation* to re*production* is telling. Conception was formerly seen as fundamentally out of the control of a person having sexual relations, and hence as a mysterious participation in *God's* act of creating a new life. Now conception is increasingly seen as something very much within our control, and hence as an expression of *human* action that produces something by our ingenuity. What then are children? Are they gifts from God to be received unconditionally, gratefully, and as ultimately our equals? Or are they products of our labor, and hence to be viewed as our possession and able to be designed and manipulated (or rejected) according to our preferences, as with other property? Conceiving, bearing, and raising children are defining aspects of human life, and a shift from seeing children as gifts of God to seeing them as products of our labor therefore promises to redefine our understanding and experience of human life. Similarly, sexual activity is a defining aspect of human life. A shift from experiencing sex as always potentially leading to pregnancy to experiencing it without that possibility promises to change the very character of sex itself. The possibility of conception heightens the stakes of sexual relations, both making marital sex more profound and putting constraints on promiscuity.

Even if Christians do not conclude that sex and procreation are absolutely inseparable, we do well to contemplate the danger of contemporary tendencies. To lose a sense of their connection will change our outlook on and experience of both sex and having children. While many in our world see this change as liberating and beneficial, Christians are right to be wary. Improving our ways of making babies is not analogous to improving our ways of making televisions. To whatever extent we proceed down the new road open before us, we certainly ought to do so cautiously.

How Many Children to Have?

Most couples at some point will consider taking action to prevent conception. This raises challenging moral questions. What theological considerations can help people begin to think through this issue?

Deciding Not to Have Children

Christians have generally acknowledged the good of having children. Against the common contemporary assumption that an expanding population is fundamentally an assault upon the earth, Christianity affirms that God meant the earth to be populated. As discussed earlier in this chapter, barrenness was a profound curse in the Old Testament, and a man with children was regarded as greatly blessed. In the New Testament barrenness is no longer treated as a curse, and there is no difference in status between being married and unmarried. Nevertheless, the New Testament hardly has a negative view of bearing and raising children. Jesus himself welcomed children warmly, teaching that "Whoever receives one such child in my name receives me, and whoever receives me, receives not me but him who sent me" (Mark 9:37). In this context Jesus was speaking about a general attitude toward children (as part of a larger point about humility), but other passages affirm the continuing goodness of bearing children of one's own. First Timothy 5:11–14 offers an interesting example. Paul first writes words similar to 1 Corinthians 7, suggesting that a widow's remarriage is not the only option and perhaps not even the ideal option. But then he concludes with the following counsel: "I would have younger widows marry, bear children, manage their households, and give the adversary no occasion for slander" (1 Tim. 5:14). Even if it is not the only acceptable way of life, having children is a good thing, and it is the course that Paul recommends for most young women, and thus necessarily for most men as well.

Most streams of the Christian tradition, however, have denied that God places an obligation upon married couples to bear as many children as possible. This is true even of official Roman Catholic teaching, despite its prohibition of all artificial methods of birth control. A number of biblical and theological considerations support this broad consensus among professing Christians.

Consider first the initial command that God placed upon the human race: "Be fruitful and multiply and fill the earth . . ." (Gen. 1:28). To interpret this as a command for all people to be maximally fruitful suffers from the fatal flaw that it brings this command into conflict with the New Testament's insistence—in 1 Corinthians 7 most notably—that choosing not to marry at all is an acceptable and even preferential decision for some Christians. It also conflicts with Paul's allowing married couples, for reasons of mutual spiritual edification, to refrain from sexual relations for periods of time (1 Cor. 7:5). How can Paul give such counsel without simultaneously revoking the creational command to be fruitful, which is repeated in Genesis 9? For one thing, the commands in Genesis 1:28 and 9:1, 7 are general imperatives given not to individuals but to the human race as a whole (through their representatives, Adam and Noah). The very fact that God commands not only being fruitful and multiplying but also *filling the earth* demonstrates that this task is not given to people individually or as married couples, but to the human race in general. In addition, it is important to remember that this creational command is stated *positively* rather than *negatively*. Negative prohibitions in Scripture are such that they are always to be observed (with certain exceptions). We are *never* to kill, to steal, or to commit adultery. But positive exhortations are often not meant to require *constant* observance. Scripture commends hard work, worship, and the training of our children, but obviously we cannot engage in all of these simultaneously. Not all biblical commands apply to all people, for different obligations fall upon children and the elderly, husbands and wives, and ministers and lay people. But even when it is clear that a positive command applies to one of us personally, the question still arises as to how much time and energy we are to devote to this particular obligation in light of our many other obligations. Clearly a person would take the obligation to pray and worship in a morally improper way if he spent so much time on these activities that he could not hold down a job or spend time with his children, leaving his household impoverished or undisciplined.

If this is true of the most important thing that we do (worship), then it certainly could be true for procreating. In other words, if it is possible to worship too much, to the detriment of one's other legitimate responsibilities, then by analogy it may be possible to be too fruitful and multiply too many times, to the detriment of other obligations. The key principle is that a married couple's procreative life ought to be carried out thoughtfully and in harmony with the full range of their responsibilities. Human beings are not bunnies in heat who simply follow their carnal impulses and deal with the consequences later. God made his image bearers morally responsible creatures who must answer for their actions. The fact that people have sexual desires, that these desires were created by God, and that they are therefore inherently good, should never be denied. But sexual desires ought to be exercised in conjunction with self-control: "For this is the will of God, your sanctification: that you abstain from sexual immorality; that each one of you know how to control his own body in holiness and honor, not in the passion of lust like the Gentiles who do not know God" (1 Thess. 4:3–5). Even our innate desires and impulses must be channeled in morally responsible directions. Each married couple, therefore, ought to be fruitful and multiply only in a way that is consistent with the other good things that God has called them to pursue.

In light of these considerations, someone may ask, how many children should a couple try to have? It is important to emphasize that this question cannot be answered! There is no single correct answer. God does not reveal in Scripture the perfect number of children for each family, and where Scripture is silent, Christians and their churches must refuse to lay binding obligations upon each other's consciences. The subject of wisdom considered at the end of the preceding chapter becomes especially crucial here. Christians must seek to grow in wisdom so that, when faced with situations where there is no universally binding answer, they will have the discernment to recognize the relevant factors and to make responsible decisions.

Considerations for Decision Making

What are some of the relevant factors that couples might take into account? What other obligations must be weighed alongside the task of procreating? One factor is financial. Among many biblical responsibilities that are financial in nature, Scripture warns us about the dangers of falling into debt (e.g., Prov. 6:1–5; 22:7). This means that it is morally legitimate for couples to consider postponing conception during times when having children would require heavy borrowing. Another financial obligation in Scripture is that parents should save for their children in order to leave them an inheritance (Prov. 13:22). There is obviously no set amount that Scripture prescribes, but the number of children that a couple has clearly affects their ability to fulfill this command responsibly. Thus we might consider a situation in which one or both spouses are pursuing further education, and they are living on a very tight budget. Having children is a good thing, avoiding debt is a good thing, and pursuing education is a good thing (among other reasons, a good education may better enable them to provide an inheritance for their children one day)—but they may not be able to pursue all of these good things simultaneously. Should they seek to have children now, or wait until they complete their academic programs? There is not one right answer for all couples in such a situation. But if a couple determines that postponing conception for a time would enable them to pursue all of these good things in the long term, while having children immediately would not, then finishing their degrees before having children is a morally sound choice.

More important than financial matters are the training, discipline, and instruction that parents owe to their children. Scripture has much more to say about how we care for our children once they are born than how many of them we should have (e.g., Prov. 22:6; Eph. 6:4).

In both bearing *and* caring for children we image God, who not only made the world in his work of creation but also sustains the world moment by moment in his work of providence. As God did not make a world that he was unable to maintain and protect, so we should not bear children to whom we are unable to give proper care. To procreate responsibly means to do so with an honest appraisal of our capability to discipline children and to raise them in the fear of the Lord. The failure to discipline and raise children well, even on the part of godly leaders like Eli, Samuel, and David (1 Sam. 2:12–36; 8:1–9; 2 Sam. 13–14), has been disastrous for God's people, and leaders of the New Testament church continue to be tested by these criteria (1 Tim. 3:4–5).

Finally (though this list is certainly not exhaustive), concern about a potential mother's health is a proper factor to weigh when considering whether to pursue procreation. God made us with bodies that reflect his own image, and the New Testament expresses concern about how we use and care for our bodies (e.g., 1 Cor. 6:19; 1 Tim. 4:8; 5:23). Pregnancy even in the best of circumstances effects significant changes in a woman's body, and having too many children in too short a space of time can have adverse effects on it. For some women, due to a variety of chronic conditions, pregnancy may mean significant physical danger to them or to their babies. The general obligation to care for our bodies, not to mention the husband's responsibility to care for his wife (Eph. 5:28), makes health a valid concern when we are faced with decisions about procreation.

It is necessary to keep these considerations in mind when pursuing the issue of morally responsible procreation. But there are also genuine dangers of abuse. The above-mentioned factors, which couples should consider, can become excuses to justify selfish, materialistic, or cowardly decisions not to have children. The financial issues offer the greatest temptation for many. While Scripture warns us about falling into debt and encourages us to save for our children, it also warns us starkly about greed and its dire consequences. Postponing pregnancy because of a desire to avoid debt is not the same thing as choosing not to have (additional) children because of fear that children would threaten our ability to maintain a lifestyle of luxury that keeps pace with our peers or neighbors. This is an excellent example of the importance of contentment. God calls us not to set our hearts on material abundance and not to avoid wholesome activities in order to pursue dreams of wealth. Paul writes: "Now there is great gain in godliness with contentment, for we brought nothing into the world, and we cannot take anything out of the world. But if we have food and clothing, with these we will be content. But those who desire to be rich fall into temptation, into a snare, into many senseless and harmful desires that plunge people into ruin and destruction. For the love of money is a root of all kinds of evils. It is through this craving that some have wandered away from the faith and pierced themselves with many pangs" (1 Tim. 6:6–10).

Along similar lines, recognizing an imminent risk of bodily harm from pregnancy or a genuine inability to care for a child that might be conceived is not the same thing as recognizing the *possibility* of bodily harm or of inability to care for a child. Whenever parents bring children into the world, there is the possibility that pregnancy might cause bodily harm to the mother, that parents—by death, illness, or accident—might become unable to care for their children, or that parents might make serious mistakes in their discipline. Here we do well to remember the virtue of courage. Having children inevitably makes a person vulnerable, liable to disappointment and grief, and at risk of financial and physical harm. If such fears are enough to justify a decision to avoid bearing children, then how would the mandate to be fruitful and multiply ever be pursued? As discussed in chapter 3, God does not call us to expunge fear, but he does call us to exercise courage in the face of genuine danger. Just as having children and thereby sacrificing a degree of opulence can be a godly expression of contentment, so having children even when afraid of the vulnerability that it brings can be a godly expression of courage, not to mention faith in the God who promises never to leave us or forsake us. There is never a perfect time to have children, if by that one means a time when parents may welcome children into the world without need to make sacrifices in their finances, careers, and friendships. To seek the perfect time for childbearing, or for any other human activity, is to seek something unattainable in this world and is inconsistent with the Christian's recognition that we cannot avoid suffering in the present life.

Moral responsibility requires more, however, than simply keeping these factors in proper perspective. We should also recognize that being in a position to bring children responsibly into this world is not something that simply happens to us. Few couples will find themselves unwittingly prepared to raise children. By doing the sorts of things that all Christians should seek to do, couples will contribute significantly to their readiness to be parents. If they learn to handle their resources with godly stewardship, to work hard at their occupations, to pursue bodily health, and to grow in wisdom and the other virtues, then they will be better equipped to welcome children with confidence that they can provide for them and train them responsibly. To avoid having children because of one's debt, when that debt is simply the result of financial irresponsibility, is surely not morally sound.

For the mutual welfare of Christians in the church, we ought to remember again that these matters do not lend themselves to clear-cut, black-and-white answers. Each married couple's situation is unique. Different couples have different financial resources, different levels of health and energy, different vocational commitments, and even different degrees of zeal for raising children. No one can know another's situation in its holistic unity, nor can one peer into another's motives. One person should not view her own experiences, struggles, and desires and assume that everyone else is identical. We do well to exhort each other to pursue the various obligations and virtues to which we are called, but we must also not be quick to judge others' decisions about having children when Scripture is silent.

Having No Children at All?

One question that sometimes arises is whether it is ever permissible to seek to have no children at all. In most cases couples that take measures to prevent pregnancy do so only for a time, with full intention of having children someday. In principle it is difficult to see why, if it is acceptable not to have children *now*, it is unacceptable not to have children *indefinitely*. Perhaps couples pondering whether they should have no children at all should be especially attentive to illegitimate rationalizations of their moral choices, but it is not difficult to think of a variety of situations in which such a decision may be legitimate. If a woman's temporary physical malady is sufficient to justify postponement of pregnancy, then a chronic, noncurable malady is surely sufficient to justify avoiding pregnancy altogether. Furthermore, while a decision to have no children because children would threaten an affluent way of life is morally suspect, other decisions to have no children based upon one's way of life deserve a different and more sympathetic moral evaluation. For example, what if one spouse is pursuing a line of work that places him or her constantly on the road or frequently in situations of physical danger? May this couple reasonably conclude that bearing and raising children responsibly is incompatible with this way of life? It is easy to imagine, of course, people pursuing such occupations for selfish or materialistic reasons, but some people do so self-sacrificially, putting their own convenience, comfort, and safety at risk in order to do benevolent work, which few others are willing to do, on behalf of the church or the broader society. Both a decision to curtail such work for the sake of having children and a decision to give up having children for the sake of continuing such work could be morally sound, and those who choose the latter route may reflect something analogous to the way of life that Paul commended in 1 Corinthians 7:32–35.

One situation that provokes the question whether to have no children at all is when a couple knows with some degree of certainty that their potential children are at great risk of a serious genetic disease. With contemporary advances in genetic technology this will likely pose more of an issue in the future than it has in the past, as medical knowledge will offer more detailed and accurate predictors of the risks involved for particular pregnancies. Here again it is probably impossible to give absolute answers that will fit each particular situation. On the one hand, declining to have children in such circumstances because one considers handicapped children to be less valuable or less worthy of love and attention than children able to lead normal lives is hardly compatible with biblical teaching. Scripture exhorts us to love the weak and helpless and gives us confidence that our handicapped children too are heirs of eternal life and blessedness. Likewise, an excessive scrupulousness about avoiding risk and vulnerability, which leads to a decision not to have children because of even a slight chance of handicap, seems incompatible with a Christian theology of suffering and courage. On the other hand, even those fully committed to loving and caring for a handicapped child, should the need arise, have morally valid reasons to consider not conceiving children. Simply because it is virtuous to respond well to a tragic situation does not necessarily mean that it is virtuous to pursue a course of action that makes that tragic situation likely to occur. And even though it is commendable for parents to endure the hardship of having a handicapped child with courage and cheerfulness, they should not be quick to impose hardship upon others. It may be that a handicapped child they produce would suffer much more than they themselves would. Couples must be very careful not to look upon their potential child as a tool for displaying their own virtue, without due consideration of the hardship that this other human person may have to endure.

Stunted Marriages?
I have suggested that there are many factors that may incline a married couple, for a brief time or perhaps even indefinitely, to take measures to avoid having children. I have also warned about the temptation to take morally valid considerations and to use them illegitimately to justify morally problematic decisions. Where does this leave couples who actively seek to prevent bearing children, in light of my reflections concerning the link between sex and procreation? Are couples who do not seek to be maximally fruitful depriving themselves of the full good of marital sexual relations? Are they falling into the contemporary mindset of placing a breech between sex and procreation, which God designed to accompany one another?

In some sense it is true that they are deprived of the full good of marital sexual relations when they do not enjoy the blessing of bearing and raising children. But in this fallen world, a world of suffering and scarcity, the dream of having it all will constantly prove to be elusive. Those who choose to chase all of the potential goods that the world offers often find themselves losing the goods that they already enjoy. Ideally, every marriage would be blessed with children—along with financial prosperity, health, and vocational fulfillment. But Christians know that they are called to suffer in this present age under the wise and loving providential hand of God. Just as the circumstances of life may compel a person to give up attempts for wealth, health, and the ideal job that would threaten other valuable goods of life, so also they may compel a person to give up, or at least to postpone, the bearing of children. Yet Christians should be comforted to know that God may still bless a couple's sexual intimacy even when it is not procreatively fruitful. First Corinthians 7:1–5 describes the good of such intimacy for the purpose of avoiding immorality, and it does so without any reference to procreation. More profoundly, the Song of Solomon celebrates sexual intimacy in terms of the delight and pleasure that it brings to the couple, and it also does so without a single reference to bearing children. By God's grace, sexual relations can fulfill God's good purposes in this fallen world even apart from the good of procreation that ordinarily accompanies it.

Method of Birth Control

When a couple seeks to postpone conception, another important bioethical question arises: are certain methods of birth control morally legitimate and others not? Again, this is an issue for which Scripture gives no explicit instructions. Some people have claimed that the story in Genesis 38 speaks to the issue. In this account God condemns Onan because he "would waste the semen on the ground" (Gen. 38:9). In context, however, it is clear that God puts him to death not because of his practice of birth control per se, but because of his refusal to fulfill his duty to raise up a child for his deceased older brother (see also Deut. 25:5–10). Since Scripture is silent on methods of birth control, we must again proceed with caution and seek to identify morally relevant considerations that can help us to make wise decisions in particular circumstances.

The first issue that should be addressed is the destruction of embryos as a method of birth control. Chapter 6 is dedicated to considering the status of human embryos, and here I assume the conclusion that I argue there, namely, that embryos are human beings and image bearers of God whose lives should be protected. If this is the case, then destroying embryos as a method of birth control is inherently wrong. This aspect of the present question requires a black-and-white answer. Such a conclusion rules out abortion as a means of birth control, of course, though presumably few people, no matter what their view of embryos, would ever look at abortion as the primary means of birth control. But it also rules out devices such as the RU-486 pill—which is specifically designed to have an abortifacient effect by blocking hormones necessary for a pregnancy to continue—and the "morning-after" pill, which may prevent pregnancy by prohibiting a fertilized egg from attaching to the uterus. This concern for the protection of the human embryo also raises questions about common birth control methods such as the oral contraceptive pill ("the Pill") and intrauterine devices (IUDs). Some writers have presented strong evidence that these methods occasionally prevent pregnancy not by prohibiting conception (their stated purpose) but by prohibiting implantation after fertilization occurs. Other writers, however, have argued that they do not have an abortifacient effect. This seems to be a question that remains scientifically disputed, and I have no scientific expertise to offer my own judgment. Whatever other considerations may contribute to a decision about use of such methods, believers concerned about the well-being of the human embryo should take this question into mind and seek the best medical counsel that they can obtain.

Within Christian circles, the main disputes about methods of birth control concern "natural" versus "artificial" means. Natural means of contraception involve refraining from sexual intercourse during periods when the woman is perceived to be fertile. The older, so-called rhythm method consists of refraining from intercourse during a certain number of days calculated from her last period. A newer method, commonly called natural family planning (NFP), operates instead by observing physical changes in the woman's body in order to determine when she is ovulating and hence susceptible to conception. The rhythm method is notoriously unreliable, if for no other reason than because women's cycles are often irregular. Conversely, many have lauded the reliability of NFP. A plethora of artificial means of contraception also exist. In one way or another these involve preventing sperm and egg from reaching each other in the aftermath of sexual intercourse.

Is there a moral difference, in principle, between using natural and artificial means of preventing pregnancy? Traditional Roman Catholicism, as affirmed by the Vatican in recent generations through famous documents such as *Humanae Vitae* and *Donum Vitae*, has posited that natural methods may be acceptable, but that all artificial means are immoral. Though some Protestants have supported this Roman Catholic position, most have accepted in principle the moral legitimacy of artificial contraception, as have many Roman Catholic theologians and laypeople. Various reasons have been offered in support of the traditional Roman Catholic position. Older arguments rested upon a teleological biology in which contraception was portrayed as prohibiting conception as the natural and proper end of the sexual act. Contemporary defenders of the position generally avoid this sort of reasoning, but argue instead that artificial contraception illegitimately prevents husband and wife from giving of themselves fully to each other in the act of sexual intercourse or that it entails acting against one of the basic human goods—that is, life—which is always inherently immoral.

In my judgment, there may be practical reasons to prefer natural over artificial methods of birth control, which I will address briefly below, but arguments that artificial methods are inherently sinful are simply not persuasive. If, as argued above, acting purposefully to avoid having as many children as physically possible can be a morally sound decision, then there is no theoretical difference between artificial and natural means of attaining this end. Even if the use of artificial contraception can be properly characterized as spouses' withholding of their full selves from each other in sexual intercourse, it is difficult to see why this is any worse than abstaining from sexual intercourse altogether during a woman's fertile period and thus withholding themselves *entirely* from each other. Even if the use of artificial contraception may be properly characterized as acting against life as a basic human good, it is difficult to see why intentionally refraining from intercourse altogether during a woman's fertile period is not just as clearly (and even more definitively) acting against the attainment of that good.

As many writers have observed, arguments that artificial contraception is inherently immoral tend to focus upon the discrete sexual act and to analyze the moral status of this act on its own terms, instead of viewing individual acts of sexual intercourse in light of the broader relationship in which they occur. Whether an individual act is theoretically "open" or "closed" to procreation seems much less significant than the broader marital relationship, given that sex within marriage, unlike most extramarital liaisons, is anything but a discrete act comprehensible apart from the profound relationship that the spouses enjoy in their lifelong commitment to each other. What is morally central for the Christian couple is not the method of birth control used in a discrete sexual encounter but their fidelity to biblical concerns about sexual purity, love for one another, and a wholesome attitude toward children as blessings from God.

Even if there is no principial or theoretical moral difference between artificial and natural means of birth control, there may nevertheless be practical reasons to choose one or the other, and these reasons may also involve morally significant decisions. NFP advocates often claim, for example, that NFP, when followed faithfully, is more effective in preventing pregnancy than the various artificial contraceptive methods. They also often assert that their method is easier on a woman's body than many artificial means, which manipulate hormones or have other possibly deleterious effects on her health, and that it benefits the spouses' relationship, since it requires mutual attentiveness to the wife's body and encourages mutual self-control. I offer no opinion on whether these claims are true, but they are at least plausible and worth consideration for couples making a decision about the right method of birth control. Factors such as effectiveness, a woman's health, and a couple's relationship are obviously matters of moral significance that those striving to act wisely will take into account.

One other issue to consider briefly in regard to method of birth control is the moral legitimacy of the various means of medical sterilization. If, as concluded above, there is no theoretical difference between so-called natural and artificial methods, then there seems to be no theoretical moral problem with sterilization either. The moral questions here are again practical rather than theoretical. Certain negative side effects are possible, and these ought to be taken into account. One distinctive feature of sterilization as a method of birth control is its ordinarily permanent character (though reversal is sometimes possible). Changing circumstances in a couple's life often change their attitudes toward certain issues. Though at a particular stage in life it might appear that bearing children would never again be a wise idea, new circumstances might cause a couple to regret such an assumption. In that sense, sterilization is a much more decisive action than temporary birth control measures, and should be undertaken with an extra degree of caution.

Conclusion

We have examined one of the chief beginning-of-life bioethical issues of past generations, the use of birth control in the face of changing cultural perspectives on sex and procreation. The believer seeking to live a wise and virtuous Christian life will necessarily look at such issues in a very different way from that of the surrounding culture. Though Scripture does not bind the Christian's conscience on many personal decisions about when and which birth control methods may be used, it does instill in believers a high regard for sexual intimacy within marriage and for the fruitfulness of such intimacy in the bearing of children. Yet it also reminds us that having children, and even marriage itself, are not the only goods worthy of pursuit in this fallen world, and that all family relations, while still important and valuable, have become relativized with the coming of Christ and our adoption into his household, the kingdom of God.

5

ASSISTED REPRODUCTION

While many married couples wrestle with whether they should take steps to prevent their sexual intimacy from resulting in pregnancy, other couples who earnestly desire pregnancy find that months and years go by without seeing that dream realized. This fallen world spawns many such ironies—what many can attain they do not want, and what many want they cannot attain—but in the case of procreation and infertility this irony produces an incalculable measure of anxiety and heartbreak.

Infertility truly causes a great sense of loss for many couples. This suffering is completely understandable in light of our human nature. God made us as sexual creatures, designed our sexual proclivities to be expressed in a loving marriage relationship, and established conception and childbearing as the ordinary fruit of the marital union. When married couples desire their mutual love to bring forth children who bear their image and whom they may love and raise together, they do nothing other than reflect the nature that God gave them. To respond to the suffering of infertile couples by offering them alternatives—such as adoption or remaining happily childless—is legitimate, but it risks being simplistic and thereby doing more harm than good. Continuing the biological link from one generation to another and experiencing the parent-child relationship that this establishes are profoundly meaningful actions. Choosing adoption over natural birth is not like choosing a different brand of bread at the grocery store when one's favorite brand is unavailable.

In light of this, infertility treatment has become a big business in the Western world. Recent statistics about the number of people pursuing infertility treatment and the costs incurred annually are rather staggering. The sorts of treatment now available to bring babies to the infertile are remarkable, from simple surgical procedures to cutting-edge technologies that remain largely experimental and in many cases extremely controversial. With these important things at stake—fundamental human instincts, large sums of money, and innovative medical technology—it is little wonder that issues surrounding assisted reproduction are among the most interesting and debated in bioethics.

I discuss matters of assisted reproduction in this chapter in the light of our broader Christian faith and life. Though some issues considered here have become significant public policy questions, our focus is on Christians' experience of infertility and their proper response to it in the light of contemporary options. Therefore I first reflect generally on infertility and the proper Christian attitude toward it. Then I discuss three broad categories of infertility treatment: those that involve a third-party parent (i.e., one who is not the husband or wife), those that maintain husband and wife as the biological parents, and finally the potentially one-parent option looming before us: human cloning.

A Theological Perspective on Infertility and Assisted Reproduction

Though assisted reproductive technology has hatched enormously difficult bioethical questions, it is unfair to jump immediately to its moral problems without first reflecting upon its accomplishments. As we saw in chapter 4, the Old Testament saints often lamented the curse of barrenness. For them it was a condition with no human remedy. The best that a barren woman could do (but inevitably with negative repercussions) was to send her maidservant to sleep with her husband. Infertility itself was incurable except by a miraculous intervention of God.

If the goal of medicine is to combat the loss of physical well-being in order to restore health and to promote human flourishing, then the development of medical means to make the infertile fertile is a great achievement of recent technology. Sometimes medicine is able to reverse infertility altogether, through relatively simple procedures (such as removing a growth on the uterus). In such cases a couple becomes able to conceive and bear children in the ordinary course of their relationship. Many other times the infertility itself is untreatable, and nothing can be done to make conception possible through sexual intercourse. But even in such cases medical technology now tells us that hope is not lost. A permanently infertile couple might still be able to have their own biological children. At the least complicated level, a husband's sperm may be inserted into his wife's body, with the goal that ordinary fertilization will occur in the fallopian tubes. At a much more complicated level, a husband's sperm and his wife's eggs may be united outside of her body. If fertilization occurs in the laboratory, the embryo can then be inserted into her body with the goal of implantation and successful pregnancy.

These technological innovations, however, open up so many other possibilities as well. The same technology that enables a wife to be inseminated with her husband's sperm enables her to be inseminated with another man's sperm. The same technology that enables a husband's sperm to fertilize his wife's egg in the laboratory enables his sperm to fertilize another woman's egg. The same technology that enables a husband's and wife's fertilized egg to be inserted into the wife's body with hope of successful pregnancy enables an egg fertilized in the laboratory to be inserted into the body of a woman who is not the biological mother. The possible scenarios are multiplying. Because sperm can be frozen and thawed with ease, a man can become a biological father many years after his death. Now that researchers are beginning to freeze and thaw eggs successfully, the same is true for women. The recent experiments with freezing young women's ovarian tissue and transplanting it back into them when they are older means that a sixty-year-old woman may be able to produce the eggs of a thirty-year-old—her own eggs, no less. And all of this pales before the prospect of human cloning, which seems technologically possible even if it has not yet been performed. Cloning offers a way not simply of making ordinary sexual relations unnecessary for successful pregnancy but even of making the union of a sperm and egg unnecessary.

May Christians participate in such things? Are there any lines in the development of reproductive technology that Christians should not cross? These questions seem to place Christians in a difficult moral quandary. On the one hand, Christians view bearing and raising children as a good thing, and therefore the general goal of reproductive technology is admirable. Furthermore, Christians ought to have a generally high view of technological progress, since it reflects our call to exercise dominion over the earth as divine image bearers. On the other hand, as discussed in chapter 4, Scripture also trains Christians to look at sex and procreation within marriage as coordinated activities. Maintaining the connection between sex and procreation protects us from viewing children as products of our own will rather than as gifts from God that are ultimately far beyond our mastery. Whether it is good to invent new and better ways of making babies is not the same moral question as whether it is a good thing to invent new and better ways of making cell phones.

Some have argued that by separating sex and procreation through artificial contraception (in other words, by promoting sex without procreation), society has inevitably opened the door wide to the disturbing scenarios made possible through assisted reproduction (in which there is procreation without sex). While it is unlikely that contemporary social approval of artificial contraception and contemporary social approval of assisted reproduction are entirely unrelated, other writers have noted that artificial contraception and assisted reproduction do not necessarily go hand in hand. In fact, the moral issues related to assisted reproduction are much more radical and profound. People have always known that sex may not lead to procreation. Experience testifies that most acts of unprotected sexual intercourse do not result in pregnancy. But the idea that procreation might be possible apart from sex was unheard of until recent years. Only by a miracle could a virgin give birth. The moral issues related to assisted reproduction are more radical and profound also because *producing* a human being is more momentous than *failing to produce* one. It makes little sense to say that a couple has wronged the (nonexistent) child that might have been born had they not used contraception. But to ask whether someone has done wrong to an existing child produced through assisted-reproductive techniques is a weighty moral question. Another weighty moral question is whether it is acceptable to subject an embryo created through artificial means to manipulation, experimentation, or disposal.

Before examining specific assisted-reproduction methods, we should examine in more depth infertility itself, the condition out of which assisted-reproduction questions arise. What is the proper Christian attitude toward infertility? If we are to look at assisted reproduction as an option that people face in the context of their broader Christian life and as a response to a particularly difficult kind of suffering, rather than as a technical, isolated, or discrete moral issue, then it is necessary first to consider infertility and the proper Christian attitude toward it. This inquiry should color our perspective on assisted reproduction itself.

Infertility and the Coming of Christ

As explored in chapter 4, God designed the marriage relationship to be one of mutual help and love with exclusive sexual intimacy. The ordinary fruit of this sexual intimacy is bearing children. In bearing children couples not only carry out the original creation mandate, as renewed in the covenant with Noah (Gen. 1:28; 9:1, 7), but also reflect the image of God, who revealed himself in Genesis 1 as a creative and fruitful God who brought new life into existence. Throughout the Old Testament, marriage and procreation took on special significance, not merely as a way of pursuing God's purposes for the human race in creation but also as a way of participating in God's redemptive promises. By having children, Israelites shared in the hope that one day the seed of the woman would crush the head of the serpent, they contributed to the fulfillment of God's covenant oath to Abraham that the number of his descendants would be like the sand of the sea, and they passed along to another generation their family's inheritance in Canaan, the pledge of an everlasting heavenly inheritance. To be unmarried was never presented as an option in the Old Testament and to be barren was reckoned a terrible curse.

In chapter 4 I also argued that the New Testament presents a striking shift in perspective. In the New Testament, remaining unmarried is an option—even a better option for some Christians. The New Testament never describes barrenness as a curse for Christians, and it does not even mention it as a source of suffering. The reason is that the virgin birth of our Lord Jesus Christ brought an Old Testament theme to dramatic climax: the barren woman has brought forth a son. The promises to Adam and Eve and later to Abraham and to Israel were all fulfilled in him. For Christians the most important parent-child relationship is their adoption as the children of God. Their brothers and sisters in the church have become closer family than their own biological relatives. Because of this, family relations, including the bearing and raising of children, are relativized in their importance for the Christian.

Yet it is hardly possible to leave things at this point, as if instructing infertile Christian couples in these truths is sufficient to wipe away suffering and to instill a brand new outlook on life. Being unable to have children (or, for some couples, being unable to have more children than they already have) brings gnawing sorrow and frustration to countless Christians. The way that God has created us makes such sorrow and frustration very natural. By God's design, nature inclines most married couples to desire their own biological children as a result of their mutual love and intimacy, and when that fails to come to fruition, a sense of profound loss is understandable and even expected.

The coming of Christ and the transformed New Testament understanding of marriage and childbearing does not change the fact that infertility means suffering, even for Christians. The reality of Christ's completed work does not change our created nature. But it is imperative for Christians to recognize that the work of Christ has called for a change in our response to the inevitable tribulations that fallen nature brings. Christ's death and resurrection have not changed the intrinsic character of death as something horrible, grief-producing, and contrary to God's original design for the human race, but they have radically changed Christians' perspective on their own experience of death. Analogously, Christ's death and resurrection call upon Christians suffering under the burden of infertility to experience their affliction in a way radically different from the way in which the world experiences it.

Infertility and Christian Virtue

One distinctive way in which Christians ought to respond to infertility is with the virtue of *contentment*. To say that Christians should be content in the face of infertility is *not* to suggest that they may never do anything to remedy their infertility. But Christians *first* ought to strive after contentment in their infertility and *only then* to consider what, if anything, to do to remedy it. This is, I believe, a crucial point to grasp if we are to respond to infertility in a way that reflects the reality of our new life in Christ. As explored in chapter 3, Christian contentment has nothing to do with attaining peace through the disappearance of all earthly problems. Instead, Christian contentment is about finding peace *in the midst of* our suffering. It is about feeling satisfaction, joy, and gratitude before God even if our problem *never goes away*. Christians are called to be content in every situation and in the face of every loss, not because a situation or a loss is insignificant or will be resolved soon, but because the abundance that God has given us in Christ brings peace and joy even in the midst of great earthly deprivation.

In the context of infertility, this means that God calls Christians to be content *in their infertility*. They must be content in *never* having any children. By God's grace, this is possible not because we should buck up and be tough, but through appreciating and giving thanks for the amazing blessing of being "members of the household of God" (Eph. 2:19). We who were once slaves under the bondage of sin have received, through the redeeming work of Christ, "adoption as sons" (Gal. 4:5). "And because you are sons, God has sent the Spirit of his Son into our hearts, crying, 'Abba! Father!' So you are no longer a slave, but a son, and if a son, then an heir through God" (Gal. 4:6–7). Paul makes the same point in Romans 8:14–17, where he makes clear that being "heirs" of our heavenly Father means nothing less than being "fellow heirs with Christ" and that therefore we have a sure hope of one day being "glorified with him." These are truly profound benefits for rebellious sinners. In conjunction with this, God has brought believers into the fellowship of the church, an assembly of the "brothers" and "sisters" called to love, serve, and encourage one another in a self-sacrificial, Christlike spirit. All of this explains Jesus' exhortation that we should be willing to give up earthly family relations for the sake of belonging to him—else we will be reckoned unworthy of him (Matt. 10:35–39). By saying this, Jesus did not suggest that it is an easy or inconsequential action. Instead, he considered this to be part of a person's "taking his cross and following me" and "losing his life for my sake." The suffering is real, but we must recognize that the blessings of adoption in Christ and of an everlasting inheritance as heirs of a heavenly kingdom far surpass the burden of suffering.

Those struggling with infertility, therefore, are called, before anything else, to find comfort and encouragement in Christ and the fellowship of his church and pray for contentment in the unearned bestowal of adoption into God's own redeemed family. I might add, in light of these things, that *all Christians*—whether unmarried or married, whether having children or not—ought to do their part, by God's grace, to make Christ's church the sort of place that does indeed provide a new and better family here and now for believers, a community that not just theoretically but in practice loves, serves, and encourages one another in whatever situation they find themselves. The church so frequently falls into the temptation, often under the pious guise of being "family friendly," to treat marriage and child-bearing as normal and singleness and childlessness as strange, and to leave the unmarried and childless either to find their own outlets for fellowship or to accommodate themselves somehow to the happy parents' child-centric forms of fellowship. If the church can resist this temptation, it will not only make the affliction of infertility much easier to bear (and in precisely the way that Christ appointed) but will also help settled Christian families to avoid idolization of their own children.

Infertile Christian couples who learn contentment in the midst of their suffering may certainly explore their options for overcoming infertility. As in all situations in which contentment is learned in the midst of suffering, however, the attainment of contentment is bound to change our outlook on the suffering itself. Because of their faith, infertile Christians know that having children is not the most important thing. They ought not to approach infertility treatment out of a sense of desperation or be willing to pay any price in order to bear their own children. Their contented, Christ-transformed perspective should enable them to consider remedies for infertility along with other godly options that may be open to them if they remain—or precisely *because* they remain—childless.

In addition to contentment, *courage* is another important virtue to cultivate in the face of infertility. Even in the age of Medicare, the prospect of facing old age without any descendants to provide support can be frightening, but Christians must beware of letting fear dictate their moral choices. Christ has brought believers into his own household, the church, and commanded his people to have special concern for the needy who lack family support (see 1 Tim. 5:3–16).

In response to their fears about enduring old age alone, Christians should remember that their Lord has established, in the community of believers, a source of care and encouragement for the needy. From the cross Christ demonstrated concern for his mother as she faced the advance of years without her eldest son (John 19:26–27). By appointing John as her "son," Jesus pointed to the benevolent character of the family of faith. As they trust in Christ's provision for his people, Christians should have the courage to face old age without children, and thus should not be overcome by fear in responding to infertility.

Christian *stewardship* is also a relevant virtue in light of the financial costs of treating infertility. According to a recent source, Americans spend over three billion dollars a year on infertility treatment. A single round of in vitro fertilization (IVF) (which frequently does not result in a successful pregnancy) costs more than twelve thousand dollars. Such numbers provoke the question whether individuals and society at large are investing these resources wisely. An immediate objection to asking such questions may arise: how can anyone place a price tag on a child? Of course one cannot put a price on a person, but that is not what the stewardship question asks people to do. When an infertile couple faces the question whether to pay twelve thousand dollars for a round of IVF (or some other amount for another infertility treatment), they cannot avoid the question whether this is the best way for them to spend this money that God has entrusted to them, in light of the other ways in which they might put that money to use. No price tag can be put on a child, but there are also many other things upon which no price tag can be placed. No price can be placed on the conversion of a sinner or the adoption of an orphaned child, for example, but that twelve thousand dollars potentially available for a round of IVF might also be used for these ends. It is important to emphasize that Christians should not expect to find a black-and-white correct answer to such stewardship questions in Scripture or anywhere else. Using the twelve thousand dollars to try a round of IVF or to support missions or to fund adoption may all be good uses of these resources. Three Christian couples in similar circumstances might make three different decisions and all of them act righteously in so doing. But each one facing such a choice is responsible before God to undertake the decision thoughtfully, wisely, and selflessly.

Responding to Infertility: What Are the Options?

With these considerations before us, what are the other options available to infertile couples besides pursuing a biological child of their own through infertility treatment? There are two principle options: adoption or remaining childless. We may consider adoption first. In order to evaluate this option properly, it is important to view adoption from a healthy perspective. It does not seem unfair to say that far too often adoption is an act of self-satisfaction or self-fulfillment. Couples who are unable to have children find an adoption agency who will provide them a healthy child of the same racial background who can come as close as possible to being the child that they themselves would have conceived had they been able. All of this is entirely understandable and not necessarily wrong. If the desire to have one's own biological children is natural and morally upright, then the desire to have what we think of as the next best thing is certainly reasonable. The adoption experience and adoptive relationship is often difficult for parents and especially children, and difficulties can be exacerbated if the child has significant health problems or is of a different racial background from the parents.

But what if we retooled our perspective on adoption, from that of fulfilling our own desires to that of self-sacrificial love? In other words, what if we looked at adoption not from the perspective of the parents' good but from the perspective of the child's good? Which party, after all, is suffering more: the infertile but otherwise prosperous couple or the truly unwanted child, left to the world abandoned or orphaned? The fact that many couples seeking to adopt healthy, racially homogeneous children spend long periods on waiting lists indicates that the children they receive are not in the strictest sense unwanted—they may be unwanted by their biological parents, but they are much in demand by prospective adoptive parents. Yet the world is filled with truly unwanted, deprived, and suffering children of a variety of racial backgrounds for whom no one needs to go on a waiting list to adopt. Adopting such a child is an option for couples able to have children as well as for those who are unable, but infertile couples are often in circumstances more conducive for this endeavor.

Such an endeavor is arduous and challenging in countless ways, and no one has an absolute obligation to undertake it. No one should manipulate another couple's guilt in order to force them to pursue this route or to condemn them if they make a different choice. But in light of the huge number of unwanted, needy children in the world and in light of the overflowing love that God displayed toward us in giving his own natural Son over to death in order to adopt rebellious sinners into his own blessed household, Christians struggling with the pain of infertility might consider this an option most worthy of consideration. It may be an option fraught with fear, but it is precisely in order to face fearful things that Christ bestows the virtue of courage upon believers.

Remaining childless altogether is the other option that presents itself to the infertile couple that chooses not to pursue treatment. Infertile couples have many profitable ways in which they can put their childlessness to good advantage. They may be financially generous and hospitable in ways that those with children cannot be. They may undertake time-intensive or even dangerous occupations that those with children would be irresponsible to undertake. As with those who are able to have children, the decision to remain childless should not be made in order to support a selfish, opulent, or materialistic way of life, but there are undoubtedly many righteous reasons that could justify such a decision.

Christians struggling with infertility should not jump into the infertility treatment industry without thinking. Most infertile couples will probably explore treatment options at some point, but they should never do so with the mindset that having their own biological children is *the* answer to their suffering. Having children is not the most important thing for Christians, and pursuing them at whatever cost— either financially or in terms of service to others—is hardly befitting to Christian profession and will in many cases lead only to greater suffering. Christians keeping these things in mind in the midst of their affliction will be better equipped to evaluate the range of infertility treatments with circumspection and wisdom.

Infertility Treatments

I should note a few points before beginning to evaluate infertility treatments from a Christian point of view. First, I cannot address every possible option, and I will not address at all the basic medical procedures that in some cases can actually cure infertility itself (i.e., they enable a couple to conceive a child naturally). Such treatments are generally not morally difficult, since they carry out ordinary purposes of medicine: restoring the body to normal, healthy functioning.

Second, I evaluate options under three basic headings: those that involve third-party parents, those that involve only husband and wife, and cloning, which involves only one parent. By pursuing the present question under these three headings, I discuss some of the most morally pertinent questions about infertility treatment, for the purpose of helping Christians to identify and to think through the important moral issues.

Third-Party-Parent Options

The first question concerns third-party-parent arrangements. A "third-party" arrangement refers to a situation in which someone other than the husband or wife is one of the biological parents or the one who carries the baby to term in her womb. Christian couples might consider one of these routes if they are concerned about transmitting a genetic disease, if the husband is unable to produce sperm, or if the wife is unable to produce eggs or to endure pregnancy.

Three basic third-party options exist. The first is artificial insemination, in which a man other than the husband contributes semen, which is then inserted into the wife's body during a fertile period with hope of ordinary fertilization and successful pregnancy. This is often referred to as "AID," since the semen comes from a donor. The second is in vitro fertilization (IVF), in which egg and sperm (one of which comes from a third-party donor) are joined in the laboratory to form an embryo, which is later inserted into the wife's body with hope of implantation in her womb. Artificial insemination and IVF can also be performed using only the husband's semen and the wife's eggs, but we will consider that later. The third situation is surrogate motherhood, in which a husband and wife contribute their own sperm and egg to create an embryo through IVF and reach an agreement with a third-party woman, the surrogate. She agrees to let the embryo be inserted into her, to carry it to term, and then to hand the baby over to the biological parents. In all of these scenarios I envision an ongoing marriage relationship and assume that the baby produced will be raised by the spouses. These procedures are in fact often used outside of marriage relationships, either by unmarried couples or unmarried individuals who wish to raise a child. I focus on scenarios that involve a marriage relationship because this book is concerned with thinking through bioethics issues in the context of the Christian life, and I thus assume the traditional biblical conviction that Christians should not cohabit in a nonmarital relationship and thus should not seek to raise a child in this context. Since AID, IVF, and surrogacy do offer the possibility of individuals producing their own biological child without a sexual relationship, some unmarried Christians may view this as a legitimate way to have children apart from marriage. We will consider this issue as well.

Couples who are contemplating one of these third-party-parent scenarios are obviously in a trying situation. They are not only unable to have children through an ordinary sexual relationship but are also unable to conceive children through the artificial joining of their sperm and egg. They have moved beyond the possibility of having children who are the biological fruit of their marital relationship. What they are contemplating, then, is a middle way: neither the biological fruit of their union nor an adopted child who is completely unrelated to them, but a child who is the biological child of *one* of them. The potential attraction of this option is understandable, for it preserves, at least in attenuated form, the strong biological link from generation to generation that serves so many important purposes. But there are serious moral problems that such arrangements create, and I conclude that though there is no explicit biblical command that prohibits third-party-parent scenarios absolutely, many reasons should deter Christians from pursuing such a course.

We may first consider third-party parent stories in Scripture in which wives give servants to their husbands in order to bear children for them. The most prominent example is that of Abraham, Sarah, and Hagar in Genesis 16, although the story of Jacob, Rachel, and Leah in Genesis 30 has many of the same elements. Like the contemporary options under consideration, in these situations the children were the biological fruit of only one spouse but were reckoned and raised as the child of both spouses (see Gen. 16:2; 30:3). Also like our contemporary options, these situations transpired with the consent of both spouses. There are also crucial differences between the biblical and contemporary situations, however. The actions of Abraham, Jacob, and their wives involved adulterous relationships and also probably involved the coercion of the servants to serve as sexual slaves. Thus these actions recorded in Scripture were *inherently immoral.*

The contemporary scenarios, which do not involve adulterous sexual intercourse and require the consent of the third-party parent, are therefore significantly different. Nevertheless, one brief observation seems relevant: harmonious family relations certainly did not result from these third-party arrangements. The story of Hagar and Ishmael was tragic, and the sons of Jacob lived in conflict and sometimes in factions. Particular dynamics attended these stories and served God's unique purposes in redemptive history, to be sure, and for this reason we should not assume simplistically that the family conflicts created in these stories will inevitably emerge in contemporary third-party-parent situations. But it is difficult not to suspect that third-party arrangements produce circumstances that are inherently dangerous for tranquil family relations.

Another biblical passage to which some have appealed for evaluating contemporary third-party-parent scenarios is Deuteronomy 25:5–10, which describes the so-called Levirate marriage. The surviving brother was to marry his dead brother's widow and to raise up children for him through her. This passage, in my judgment, is even less analogous to contemporary cases and yields no helpful insight. While there was a third party of sorts present here (the dead brother, whose child the baby is reckoned to be), the surviving brother and the widow were to marry each other, to produce the child through an ordinary marital relationship, and presumably to raise the child together. Thus, though such arrangements existed by divine ordination (unlike those of Abraham and Jacob), they do not resemble contemporary cases in any relevant detail.

Though there are no direct biblical instructions on third-party parenthood, the implications of the seventh commandment are weighty for grappling with this moral question. Some writers have posited that AID and other third-party-parent arrangements constitute an act of adultery, insofar as the presence of the third party intrudes upon what ought to be the exclusive domain of husband and wife. This is obviously a serious charge, and it merits attention. In our ordinary speech, as well as in biblical language, "adultery" refers specifically to sexual relations between a married person and someone who is not his or her spouse. Ordinarily the other spouse does not give consent, though this is not technically required for the act to be labeled as adultery. The common statement that an adulterer "cheated on" his or her spouse illustrates this presumed lack of consent. In these two important senses, therefore, the third-party parent options under consideration here are not adulterous, for they do not involve sexual relations outside of marriage, and they do require the consent of all the parties involved. These reasons alone seem sufficient to discourage use of the term "adultery" to describe them, since the term connotes the presence of sins that the spouses may have been scrupulous to avoid and prejudges the moral question in an unhelpful and unjust way.

But this does not mean that there is no relevant moral insight in thinking of third-party parenthood in terms of the seventh commandment. For though we do not ordinarily consider the presence of adulterous semen in the body of a woman or the growth of an adulterously conceived baby in the womb of a woman as themselves ongoing acts of adultery, we would certainly view these as radically out of place and as a continuing presence of the adulterer intruding into the marriage relationship. What husband would not be troubled, even after the act of adultery itself, by the thought of another man's semen in his wife's body or another man's baby growing in her womb? It is now scientifically possible for us to separate sexual intercourse from procreation and pregnancy. But apart from medical intervention, keeping sexual intimacy an exclusive matter between husband and wife necessarily means that any semen, any fertilized egg, any implanted embryo, and any growing baby in a woman's body will belong to her husband alone. God made us, therefore, with a natural understanding that not only the brief act of sexual intercourse belongs only between a husband and a wife but also that the entire process of the nine months of pregnancy is exclusive marital domain. Simply because we are able to bypass the initial step or two, thereby preserving these steps from third-party intrusion, does not mean that we are able to eradicate God-engrained desires for marital exclusivity beyond coitus. Even if both husband and wife were able to suppress whatever natural feelings of guilt and anger may arise in the aftermath of a third-party conception, it does not mean that they should, or that their relationship would remain undamaged. Our contemporary social and political milieu tends to glorify consent as the overriding test of an act's morality and legality, but Christians should not be so foolish as to think that what they consent to cannot harm them and others.

These observations perhaps do not constitute a tight moral argument against all third-party parenthood that will be immediately persuasive to all people. But even if these observations fall short as a conclusive argument and do not yield dogmatic moral rules, they demand careful Christian reflection. The institution of marriage today has been so badly damaged by adultery, the prevalence of pre-marital sex, readily accessible pornography, and easy divorce and remarriage that we should be on our guard about becoming calloused to the profundity of marital exclusivity and the subtle deleterious effects of nonexclusivity in the marital relationship. Christians ought to welcome third parties into the process of producing and bearing children only after careful and honest reflection on their commitment to their spouses in terms of the seventh commandment.

In addition to the seventh commandment, a couple of other issues raise serious concerns about third-party-parent arrangements. The first picks up on the observation regarding third-party parenthood in Genesis: third-party parenthood tinkers with family relationships in morally problematic ways. I have already reflected on the significance of biological ties between parent and child from generation to generation. In countless ways it matters who our parents and grandparents are. It matters who our children and grandchildren are. Knowing from whose loins we have sprung intimately defines our self-identity, our sense of belonging, and our perception of continuity with the past. The actions of many adopted people illustrate the fact that knowing who our *biological* ancestors are is deeply meaningful. When a person learns that he is adopted (especially if he learns it later in life), the news often affects him deeply and even traumatically. Many adopted people wish to learn who their biological parents are, even if they have been raised in a stable home by loving adoptive parents. They feel that they will not know fully who they themselves are if they do not learn about their biological heritage. In addition, we should not underestimate the personal toll that the surrogate mother may suffer in giving up the baby she has borne. Many writers have explored the various bonds created between a mother and her baby during pregnancy. The occasional story about a mother who abandons her newborn child tends to shock us as something horrific and truly *unnatural*. We are not shocked, therefore, by the fact that surrogate mothers sometimes change their minds and refuse to hand over the babies they have delivered. Signing a contract cannot wipe out bonds that are innate to human beings.

The moral question that faces us, then, is whether we ought intentionally to create situations in which biological links between generations are attenuated, confused, or even ruptured. In essence, third-party-parenthood arrangements intentionally create adoption scenarios. In the previous section I praised adoption as a charitable act that rescues abandoned and orphaned children. Surely it is a charitable act—precisely because we recognize these children's tragic circumstances. In an ordinary adoption situation the adoptive parents are *responding* to a child's tragic situation and seeking to bring good out of it. In a third-party-parent arrangement, however, the parents are *creating* a child's tragic situation, a situation in which he will be taken away from his birth mother or be raised by someone other than his biological mother or father. Or perhaps the third-party parent plans to stay involved with the child. This case is similar to the situation of a child of divorced parents who splits time between two homes and two families. Few would consider this divorce scenario to be anything other than a tragic situation and an attempt to make the best of it—certainly not something that one would wish for a child. We can therefore again conclude that Christian conviction demands the greatest caution before proceeding with third-party parenthood. Christians ought to acknowledge and cultivate the natural bonds between parents and children, not to contribute to present cultural trends that are weakening them. If a Christian couple is willing to raise a child whose natural, biological bonds have been severed, then I suggest that there should be a preference in favor of *rescuing* a child already in this situation rather than *creating* a child to be in it.

A final consideration casting doubts on third-party parenthood is the issue of commodification. Third-party-parent arrangements require, in some manner or another, the alienation (in the economic sense) of one's procreative assets. Whether it is sperm, an egg, or a womb, a part of one's reproductive system is bought and sold, donated and received, or rented or loaned. The baby-making business is already a huge international endeavor, with sperm and egg for a single child sometimes acquired from different countries (often because of different rules regulating their distribution from nation to nation). Should sperm and egg be sold on the open market like bread or cars? Should wombs be rented on nine-month leases like an apartment (or, since surrogate mothers make a whole-body commitment during the pregnancy—agreeing to eat well, to stop smoking, to refrain from certain sexual activities, and the like—perhaps the better analogy is selling one's body into tempo-rary slavery)? Intelligent writers have argued both sides of the question, and I leave it to each reader to make a judgment about the question as a public policy matter. But Christians, who view the human body as reflecting the image of God, should at least be cautious about involving themselves in procedures that treat body parts and embryos like common commodities that are bought and sold.

Let us also briefly consider whether unmarried Christians, who have a special love for children but adhere to the traditional Christian prohibition against extramarital sexual relations, might pursue AID or IVF as a legitimate way to produce children that they intend to raise as single parents. Such an action would obviously not implicate the participants in compromising the exclusivity of a marriage relationship. But if there is a God-ordained, natural connection between sexual intercourse and the development of a child in a woman's body, such that third-party parenthood threatens to compromise the exclusivity of the marriage relationship, then serious questions also arise whether unmarried people sully their sexual purity by engaging in IVF or AID. To put it in another way, if seventh-commandment purity *within* marriage extends beyond mere abstinence from sexual intercourse with someone other than one's spouse, then seventh-commandment purity *outside of* marriage arguably extends beyond mere abstinence from all sexual intercourse and includes all of a person's procreative life.

We have seen that third-party-parenthood arrangements threaten to damage important biological family relations, and many of the same problematic issues also exist in the context of an unmarried person who seeks to have a child through AID or IVF. But an additional issue exacerbates the difficulties. The unmarried person would not only create an adoptive situation but also intentionally bring a child into a single-parent home. Living in a single-parent home is never an ideal situation for a child. In most circumstances it is much better for an orphaned or abandoned child to be adopted and raised by a single parent than by no one at all, but creating a child intentionally for the purpose of being raised by a single parent is an entirely different matter. If an unmarried person is truly desirous and capable of raising a child as a single parent, a situation that will always be far less than ideal, then a strong moral presumption favors adopting a child already in a desperate situation rather than creating a child of one's own.

Husband-Wife-Only Options

Husband-wife-only options are assisted-reproduction choices that involve only the husband's semen and the wife's egg and womb. Specifically in view here are IVF and artificial insemination (here referred to as AIH, since it is the *husband's* semen which is inserted into the wife's body). These options are the most defensible means by which assisted reproduction can be undertaken, though challenging moral obstacles exist here as well, particularly for IVF.

That these husband-wife-only options are morally superior to those that involve a third-party parent is evident simply by noting how many of the ethical concerns raised above in regard to third-party arrangements are irrelevant in the present case. When husband and wife alone are involved, the seventh commandment questions need not be asked, since the exclusivity of the marital relationship is preserved through the entire process of pregnancy. Similarly, in a husband-wife-only scheme skewed biological family relations are not at stake, because the biological ties between generations are wholly preserved and no birth mother is required to relinquish the fruit of her womb. Finally, concerns about participating in the commodification of procreation are substantially lessened, since there is no need for a third party to buy or to sell some aspect of his or her reproductive life. Thus these husband-wife-only arrangements present a considerably different moral question from that of third-party-parent arrangements.

This does not mean, however, that there are no important moral questions to ask. Some voices in the broader Christian world, particularly Roman Catholic, have asserted that any method that separates ordinary marital sexual relations from the procreative process is to be avoided. As this general principle forbids all artificial contraception, so it also forbids AIH and IVF, even when no third-party parent is involved. Christian conviction about the way in which God created us offers compelling reason to respect the connection between sex and procreation and to think that ordinarily the two should be experienced in tandem. As argued in chapter 4, however, a married couple can maintain this connection in the broader course of their marriage relationship without seeking to maximize the number of children that they produce and without avoiding all contraceptive practices. If there is no moral necessity for every act of sexual intercourse to seek pregnancy as its goal, then there likewise seems to be no moral necessity for the union of a couple's sperm and egg to be linked to a specific act of sexual intercourse. Ordinarily, a couple's use of contraception is most morally attractive when it occurs in the midst of a broader marriage relationship that seeks to be procreatively fruitful in the longer term. Such a relationship continues to value the link between sex and procreation and refuses to despise the latter while enjoying the former. Along similar lines, a couple's use of assisted-reproduction methods (without third-party parents involved) is most morally attractive when it occurs in the midst of a broader marriage relationship that is sexually intimate (even if that intimacy itself cannot result in pregnancy) and thus continues to value the link between sex and procreation and refuses to despise the former while pursuing the latter.

In my judgment, there is nothing inherently immoral in a married couple's pursuing husband-wife-only assisted reproduction, so long as this link between sex and procreation is honored. But do any moral difficulties plague AIH or IVF? In the case of AIH I do not believe any such difficulties exist. When AIH is performed and the results are successful, a baby is conceived in the wife's body and develops just as if ordinary intercourse had resulted in fertilization. Even when AIH is performed and is not successful, the result is no different from any ordinary act of intercourse that does not result in pregnancy. In light of this, and in light of the relative ease and reasonable financial costs of AIH, when a married couple decides to pursue assisted reproduction, AIH seems to be the morally preferable option if it is viable.

Unfortunately, a number of moral difficulties prohibit such an easy moral approval of IVF. IVF is an immensely more complicated procedure than AIH, and its intricacies raise interrelated questions about the significant financial costs of the procedure, the health of the potential mother, and especially the treatment of the embryos created in the laboratory. In the discussion that follows I argue that there are some circumstances in which IVF should certainly not be performed, other circumstances in which considerations of wisdom offer strong reasons not to pursue it, and only limited circumstances in which it is not morally problematic. I am assuming that human embryos are image bearers of God, which ought to be cared for and protected, a position that I defend in the next chapter.

Many of the important moral questions are driven by IVF's high cost and relatively low success rate. Not all eggs that are extracted from a woman will be fertilized, and not all successfully created embryos, when inserted into the woman's body, will implant in her uterus and come to term. The probability of any single egg being fertilized, implanting in the uterus, and coming to term is low. Hence, in order to avoid the need for multiple attempts with their escalating costs, IVF clinics ordinary recommend that the woman's ovaries be artificially stimulated in order to produce multiple eggs all at once. Then practitioners extract those many eggs and join them with the husband's sperm, with the hope that some of them will be fertilized. But because *many* eggs are exposed to the sperm (in order to increase the odds of at least one fertilization), a number of viable embryos often become available. According to common practice, three or four of the embryos are then inserted into the woman's body, with the hope that one or two will implant and proceed through a healthy pregnancy. Should all of the embryos implant, abortion of all but two is usually recommended. The reasoning behind such abortions is that it is better to have two normal, healthy babies than to have all of them die in an over-crowded womb or be born prematurely with the many health risks that that entails. The embryos that are not used to attempt pregnancy are either disposed of or frozen. Those that are frozen may be used at a later point if the first attempt at pregnancy fails or if the couple desires more children.

This typical IVF procedure creates a host of moral difficulties for those who believe that an embryo is a human person and an image bearer of God. In an understandable bid to minimize costs and to maximize odds of successful pregnancy, IVF practitioners commonly seek to create large numbers of embryos. If they turn out to have more than needed, either outside or inside the womb, then some of them are destroyed. What moral constraints does this place upon Christians considering IVF?

First, all IVF procedures that make destruction of embryos an option built into the plan of action are clearly forbidden. To put this point positively, Christians may only consider pursuing IVF procedures for which they are committed to nurturing every one of their created embryos through the entire course of a pregnancy. This means that they should attempt to fertilize only as many eggs as they are committed to inserting into the wife's body, *at least at some point*, in case all of the eggs are successfully fertilized. This also means that, in any given attempt, they should insert into the wife's body only as many embryos as she can safely bring to term, in case all of them successfully implant. Hence, they should probably implant two, or at most three, in order to ensure good prospects for both the woman's health and the embryos' *in utero* flourishing. This also means, finally, that whatever embryos are created beyond the two or three that are inserted at a given time must be frozen until a later point, at which time they should be thawed and inserted into the wife's body in another attempt at pregnancy.

In my judgment, Christians must observe *at least* these constraints. Otherwise they proceed by treating the destruction of embryos as a viable option if things do not go precisely as planned. It must be noted that Christians who abide by these constraints may increase the financial and physical costs of IVF substantially. Because they will attempt to fertilize fewer than the recommended number of eggs during each round and insert fewer than the recommended number of embryos at a time, their odds of successfully carrying babies to term with each round of egg extraction is significantly reduced. This often necessitates more attempts at egg extraction, more attempts at egg fertilization, and more attempts at pregnancy for the Christian couple wishing for the birth of babies through IVF. All of this means a greater physical toll on the woman and higher financial expenses.

Considerations of wisdom add additional moral constraints to the Christian weighing IVF as an option: though freezing embryos for future use is not morally prohibited per se, freezing embryos opens the door to potential tragedies that are generally wise to avoid. I argued previously that couples who have more embryos than can be safely inserted at a given time should freeze them in order to preserve them for a future attempt at pregnancy. The intention to use the embryos later respects their status as human persons and is morally sound. In many cases couples will be able to act upon this intention. The thawed embryos will be inserted into the woman's body and may survive and be brought to term. However, no matter how pure a couple's intentions are, no couple can know with certainty that they will be able to act upon their intentions. A woman may die or become physically impaired, thus making the insertion of the thawed embryos into her body impossible. In other cases the couple's situation will change significantly—perhaps the husband dies, or the wife develops health problems that make pregnancy dangerous, or they encounter great financial hardship. Going through with their intended pregnancy, while still technically possible, comes to appear as a profound hardship or as a foolish act rather than as an exciting opportunity. To put the matter briefly, is it morally wise for a couple, who are committed to bringing to term all embryos that they create, to freeze embryos for a later day, thereby opening up the possibility that they will either not be able to use them or be able to use them only under great duress?

At this point the reader might object and point out that if *possibilities* of strange occurrences in the future must constrict our present choices then people should never have babies at all. Any parents could die in a car crash or become bankrupt six months after their baby's birth. This objection has an initial plausibility, but it is ultimately unpersuasive. Biblical wisdom certainly requires reflection upon the possibilities that might follow upon our actions. Rarely do we know with certainty what consequences will follow the acts that we perform. Proverbs 27:12 thus counsels: "The prudent sees danger and hides himself, but the simple go on and suffer for it." The fact that a couple might die shortly after their child is born does not mean that they should have no children, but means that they should take steps to ensure that someone trustworthy will adopt their child if such tragedy does strike. But then this raises the question of whether something analogous might be possible for the IVF situation. Would it be morally upright for a couple to freeze their embryos as long as they secure a commitment from another woman that she will attempt to carry these embryos to term if they become unable to do so (which is in fact an option that some Christian couples pursue)? This seems to be the only scenario in which freezing embryos might possibly be justified as a morally wise action. Nevertheless, it is probably not wise for most women in most circumstances to promise to undertake such a task (and hence not wise for most prospective parents to extract such a promise). The pledge to bear someone else's children is weighty, and no woman knows what her own future holds.

I concluded earlier that Christian couples should have only as many eggs fertilized as they are committed to using *at some point*. But if these latter reflections about freezing embryos are sound, then generally Christian couples should have only as many eggs fertilized as they are committed to using *immediately*. This means that Christians pursuing IVF should ordinarily allow no more than two eggs to be extracted and made subject to fertilization at any given time. Such a decision makes the odds of successful pregnancy for each round of IVF—each round being very expensive—rather low. My conclusion, therefore, is that, under a limited set of circumstances, IVF is a morally legitimate option. At the same time, even under these ideal circumstances, the financial and physical costs, weighed against the probability of success, require Christians to consider carefully the stewardship issues discussed earlier.

Human Cloning

Human cloning is one of the most intriguing and bizarre matters of the present day. As things stand at the time I am writing, human cloning is more of a public policy debate than a solution that individual Christians might consider for their own infertility struggles. But I give it some brief attention, since many Christians wonder about the puzzling moral implications of the yet-to-be-realized prospect of human cloning. Given that the life of human embryos should be protected, I simply assume here that human embryos should not be created through cloning in order to produce pluripotent stem cells or for other research purposes. Therefore, I discuss cloning only as an assisted-reproduction issue: how might Christians evaluate the moral propriety of cloning for the purpose of bringing a child into the world? While there is no explicit biblical guidance on the question, a number of considerations suggest a decidedly negative appraisal of this prospect.

Many readers are probably familiar with the basic facts about human cloning. Somatic cell nuclear transfer, the method used by Ian Wilmut to produce the famous cloned sheep, Dolly, would involve several steps. First the entire DNA nucleus from a woman's egg must be removed, and a cell from the person to be cloned must be brought back to a predifferentiated state. Then the DNA nucleus from this cell must be placed into the enucleated egg, thereby creating a human embryo. This embryo would then be inserted into a woman with the goal of implantation and successful pregnancy.

One initial question about cloning that some Christians have raised is whether a cloned person would have a soul. I see no good theological reason to conclude that a clone would be soulless. How the soul originates in each new human being is a theological mystery. Christian theologians have proposed two basic theories: creationism (claiming that God creates each new human soul directly, either at conception or shortly thereafter) and traducianism (claiming that the soul is propagated in the physical process of the union of sperm and egg). Neither of these theories can be proven definitively from the teaching of Scripture. In my judgment, therefore, it would be nonbiblical speculation to assert

that there is something about the formation of the embryo in the cloning procedure that obstructs the appearance of a soul. Furthermore,
the idea that there might be a living, breathing human body without a
soul seems to be a theological fantasy. According to traditional Christian theology and the teaching of Scripture, a human body without a
soul is precisely the definition of a corpse.

As an act of assisted reproduction, cloning is in a different ball-
park altogether in comparison with other options. It is a *one person* reproductive endeavor and hence entirely individualistic and
asexual. It does not merely change the circumstances in which a
sperm and egg are united but dispenses with this union altogether.
Given what I have already argued, the fact that God made us as
sexual creatures and as sexually reproducing creatures, and that
he instilled profound meaning in these aspects of human nature,
should make us suspicious of attempts to bypass them. Cloning
is more than a minor tinkering with human existence as we have
always known it.

We might also ask why a person would choose cloning as a method
of reproduction. Are there morally sound reasons to choose *this* route?
Perhaps someone would make this choice because of an exalted view
of his own genetic makeup, such that he would not wish to soil it by
mixing it with another person's? That seems to be a motive driven by
ungodly hubris. Or perhaps someone would choose cloning because
she spurns marriage and thinks that she can raise a child well without it? That could obviously not be a morally sound motive for a
Christian. Or perhaps someone would choose cloning from a desire
to live his own life all over again, as it were, through a proxy who is
genetically identical to him? That seems to make the child his tool
or property, a means for fulfillment rather than a gift. God entrusts
children to parents to raise and to train, not to control. Or perhaps a
parent would choose to clone not herself but her dead child, in order
to replace the child that was lost?

This last question encourages us to consider also how the act of
cloning should be interpreted from the clone's perspective. What
would it be like to live as a clone? One answer is that being a clone
would mean living with a very confused set of family relations. In
fact, the confusion caused by cloning dwarfs the confusion caused
by third-party parenthood situations. The same person would be the
clone's mother and identical twin. Her aunts and uncles would also

be her siblings. When she turns twenty, her stepfather might look at her and see the girlfriend of his youth. If biological family relations are important and confusing them is dangerous, then the clone's predicament would be tragic. What kind of experience would it be to see one's own genetic twin decades down the road, or to live one's life as the genetic substitute for a dead sibling? Of course no one knows exactly what this would be like or what its effects would be, but for this very reason it is not an experience that we should lightly place upon another person.

One other matter is worth brief observation: if cloning is ever to work, researchers must do extensive experimentation on human embryos. The scientists who produced Dolly the sheep failed a great many times before succeeding. How much experimentation with human embryos is morally permissible, and are we willing to risk producing people with genetic abnormalities (as was the case with Dolly) in our quest to perfect the cloning process? These are additional reasons for Christians to be skeptical of this venture.

In short, despite the Bible's obvious silence on the cloning question, numerous considerations raise pressing ethical questions about cloning as a method of reproduction. Christians seem to have good reason to resist the temptation to look to it as a promising method for the future, and they should certainly consider how they might contribute to present public policy discussions about it.

Conclusion

We have carefully considered infertility, a tragic situation in which many Christians find themselves. Though modern medicine offers innovative hope to infertile couples, it often does so with many subtle or overt costs of its own. Christians may explore modern infertility treatments, but they should be wary about pursuing many of them. In the larger picture, Christians should not begin with medicine and then turn to their faith only for succor when medicine fails, but should begin with the great truths of the faith that bring profound encouragement to the infertile whether or not they avail themselves of the options that medicine offers. While Christians continue to prize marriage and children as God-ordained gifts, the work of Christ has brought us into the church, the very household of God, and into relationships with God and our fellow believers that far transcend temporal family relations. In Christ we should face infertility not out of despair and desperation, but as those who have a hope far surpassing what fickle medicine can offer and who have opportunities for charitable acts that make infertility treatment only one of many viable options. By facing infertility with courage, contentment, and self-sacrificial charity, Christians present a witness to the world that their hope lies far beyond the passing things of this age.

6

THE HUMAN EMBRYO

When dealing with a variety of beginning-of-life bioethical issues, such as contraceptive methods and in vitro fertilization, valuing the life of the human embryo, even from its earliest days, puts significant moral constraints upon the Christian's options for preventing pregnancy and treating infertility. Therefore, it is crucial to consider several important questions: When does human life begin, and is this the same point at which human life must be protected from destruction? Does Scripture answer this question, and what sort of obligations does its teaching place upon Christians? The answers to such questions should not only underlie our attitude toward contraception and assisted reproduction but should also shape the way in which Christians participate in public policy controversies such as abortion and stem-cell research.

First we will consider what constitutes a human being and a human person (and whether there is any difference between the two), looking particularly at what a Christian theology of the image of God contributes to this question. Second, against this background, I will identify what the human embryo is, from fertilization through its development in the womb, and discuss how this developing being should be treated. Finally, we will consider the implications for abortion and stem-cell research. My general claim is that biblical, theological, and even scientific considerations, taken together, present a strong case for affirming that human embryos, beginning at fertilization, are image bearers of God whose lives are to be protected and cultivated.

Human Beings, Human Persons, and the Image of God

Many recent discussions about the status of the human embryo in theological, philosophical, and public policy settings have centered around the question of what a human *person* is. Why has this issue been so important? A little background is helpful for answering this question. At some level there is little debate that the human embryo, from its earliest days, is human life. The embryo is obviously alive, and it is clearly not some kind of life other than human. It possesses human DNA and, unless death interrupts the process, it develops in the womb, is born a human baby, and proceeds through the stages of human existence. But Western society has hotly debated whether human life in every form should be granted full human rights. This is where the issue of *personhood* becomes especially pertinent. Many writers have argued that not all living human entities are in fact human persons. Furthermore, according to this argument, only those that are persons are able to possess rights, such as the basic right to life. In light of this claim, many controversies about subjects like abortion have revolved around the definition of personhood and thus about which living human entities are persons with rights.

The answers have differed. Some parties, especially those with so-called pro-life leanings, have argued for a view of personhood that centers around genetic identity. According to this line of thought, having a human nature or a human genetic code secures one's identity as a human person. This means that even newly fertilized embryos, because their nature and genetic code are undeniably human, possess a right to life. This perspective also has implications for end-of-life issues such as euthanasia, for it entails that people who are severely disabled or in a vegetative state must also be protected as human persons. Other parties, usually associated with so-called pro-choice positions, define human personhood not in terms of human nature but in terms of actions and relationships with others. Human persons, they explain, are beings who think, make choices, and bear account- ability for those choices. Human persons are social creatures whose identity depends upon having relationships with other people. Beings that are incapable of reasoning and willing and who lack the ability to enjoy social relationships cannot be accorded full human rights. Many writers who support this sort of view also argue that nonpersons with a human nature, such as embryos or those in a persistent vegetative state, may be worthy of some respect as potential or former human persons, but not the right to life in a full sense. Others do not even make this concession, however, but relegate pre-personal human life to a status equal to or even less than that of animal life.

Given the stakes of these debates, Christians are compelled to consider what their own perspective ought to be. The notion of personhood is not foreign to Christian theology. Many of the most important affirmations of early Christian theology were tied to an understanding of "person": the church confessed that it worshiped one God who is three persons and that the Lord Jesus Christ is one person with two natures. Nevertheless, Scripture itself does not define what a "person" is, nor does it use such terminology in teaching about the Trinity or the incarnation. The church's Trinitarian and christological affirmations, crucial and true as they are, were conclusions that theologians derived from the teaching of Scripture without limiting themselves to explicit biblical language. These observations are relevant for our consideration of human personhood. We may well be able to use the term "person" in a helpful way, but if we are to discover a view of the human embryo demanded by our commitment to Christian faith and life, then we should first examine how Scripture does address the issue. The terms in which Scripture speaks are not those of human life/human personhood distinctions, but those of the image of God and what that entails.

Chapter 2 explored in some detail what Scripture teaches about the image of God. In terms of the debates over personhood, one significant fact to note is that Scripture describes the image in terms of nature, actions, and relationships. In other words, all of the chief contemporary proposals for what constitutes human personhood touch upon aspects of a holistic Christian theology of the image. Yet a full understanding of the image cannot be reduced to one or another of these aspects. The biblical outline of the doctrine can be summarized in a few points. First, the image of God entails having a certain nature. Human beings do not simply possess the image of God, but *are* the image of God. They are the image not only in soul but also in body. Their rational, volitional, and moral attributes all contribute to their image-bearing nature. The various things that Scripture says about the image—concerning knowledge, righteousness, and holiness, concerning our moral responsibility and accountability, and concerning dominion over creation—are inconceivable apart from a nature that possesses reason and will and that exists bodily without being reduced to the physical. Second, the image consists in the relationships that human beings enjoy. The image primarily involves a relationship of responsibility and accountability before God, who made us in his image to carry out the royal task of exercising dominion over the earth. In addition, God made us male and female, as beings designed neither to exist alone nor to reflect his likeness as solitary individuals, but as a community that must answer to him corporately as well as individually. Third, the image of God consists in carrying out certain tasks. The office of image bearer is a call to an active life of imaging the God who reveals himself in Genesis 1:1–25 as the one who formed and fashioned this world. To exercise dominion under God requires hard work, careful study, technological innovation, and the implementation of the various capacities that God has given to us.

In light of the matters considered in chapter 2, an image bearer is worthy of the highest respect among all of God's creatures. The image bearer is the pinnacle of creation, destined not just for life in this age but even for everlasting, heavenly life in the age to come.

What do these insights contribute to the question of when a being that possesses human life is indeed a human person, that is, a being that is owed full human dignity and protection? These theological parameters leave no doubt that a normal, healthy, mature adult is an image bearer, but that is not a point of controversy in contemporary debates. The real difficulty is applying the theology of the image to those, like newly fertilized embryos, who lack some of the characteristics that constitute the image in its fullness. What are the consequences of lacking some of the features that Scripture associates with the image of God? Must a being possess *all* of the characteristics that constitute the image in order to be an image bearer, or should those who manifest *some* of the characteristics also be reckoned as image bearers?

The answer is certainly the latter: being an image bearer does not require the manifestation of all of the characteristics of image bearing. Looking at obvious cases from adult life (rather than moving immediately to the murkier case of embryonic life) offers evidence for this claim. Since the body is part of what constitutes the image of God, then having legs is an aspect of the image. But no one would seriously suggest that a person whose legs are amputated ceases to be an image bearer. Indeed, in an analogous situation, those who are unable to walk are the subject of special human compassion in the New Testament, and Jesus declares a paralyzed man's sins forgiven (Luke 5:17–26), an incomprehensible act if this man did not bear the image. The continuing possession of other image-bearing attributes evidently ensures that people in these situations retain the status of an image bearer. Likewise, no one would seriously argue that a person who is abandoned on an island with no human companion ceases to bear God's image. Such a person may never again exercise relationships with other human beings, yet he retains other characteristics that sustain him as an image bearer. The same might be said even for a person who is sleeping. Harming a sleeping person is no less wrong than harming someone who is awake, yet a sleeping person actively exercises no relationships with others, does not exercise human dominion over the world, and does not make rational choices.

These initial considerations support the conclusion that possessing some, even if not all, of the range of characteristics that constitute the holistic image of God is sufficient to establish a human being as an image bearer. This suggests that if the embryo manifests even some of the characteristics of an image bearer then it bears the image of God and is due all of the respect that that entails.

Another initial consideration supporting this conclusion is the fact that human beings are always in the process of development. Our mental and physical abilities, as well as our abilities to experience relationships, are constantly growing or declining. Consider rationality as an aspect of image-bearing. Different people possess different degrees of rationality, and each individual person experiences increasing rationality through childhood and often declining rationality in old age. The same is true concerning our volitional attributes and our moral accountability. There is no single rational, volitional, or physical ideal. Even if we were able to identify the peak manifestation of a certain human attribute, it remains true that our various attributes peak at different times. A person often reaches her physical peak in her twenties, but attains her peak of moral competence significantly later. Furthermore, the various image-bearing attributes that a person manifests at any given time are rooted in and have been shaped by earlier stages in her development. Her capacities to think rationally, to choose morally, to execute physical skills, and to have relationships are all the product of years of formation and practice. In all of these cases, the development of these attributes began at least in early childhood, and even *in utero*. A person cannot sufficiently explain his relationship with his mother in adulthood without recognizing that the relationship forged during nine months in the womb has shaped their present relationship.

What relevance is this for the present subject? The reality of human life as we know it and our theology of the image of God mean that being an image bearer involves a variety of human characteristics in a constant flux of development and decline, of not-yet-realized potential and already-realized loss. Those who claim that performing certain human tasks and enjoying certain human relationships are requisite for being a human person thus face some difficult problems. To what degree does someone have to perform and enjoy them in order to be considered a human person? And if this long process of becoming who I am now derives back to my early childhood and even into my development in the womb, identifying a certain point in the midst of that process as the point at which personhood begins seems impossible. If my experience earlier in the process shapes my present experience of personhood, then how can that earlier experience itself not be an experience of personhood? At the very least, being an image bearer of God must be pushed back beyond early childhood into prenatal development. Whether this means all the way back to fertilization is a question that I postpone for the moment. At this point I turn to explore specific biblical teaching about prenatal human life and to show how it concurs with these general implications of our theology of the image of God.

The Biblical Perspective on Prenatal Human Life

Many studies have mined Scripture in order to identify the biblical doctrine of the origin of human personhood. Abortion is the pressing issue that has often prompted such studies. Scripture never addresses the issue of abortion itself, nor does it engage in specific doctrinal teaching on the status of the embryo. While these facts suggest that we should be cautious about coming to dogmatic conclusions too hastily, they do not mean that Scripture has nothing to say about how God views unborn human beings or about how we should treat them. My conclusion, similar to that of many other Christian writers on this subject, is that Scripture does teach that the unborn human being is an image bearer of God and should be viewed with the respect and dignity that is due to other human persons.

Writers have often turned to the Psalms to support this conclusion. Psalms 51 and 139 are of special interest since both speak explicitly about life in the womb and about the unborn human being's standing before God. Psalm 51, a well-known confession of sin, is David's prayer to God after committing adultery with Bathsheba, as recorded in 2 Samuel 11. David states: "Behold, I was brought forth in iniquity, and in sin did my mother conceive me" (Ps. 51:5). This language indicates that the psalmist is reflecting on human life from its earliest beginnings in the womb. For accuracy's sake it should be noted that the Hebrew word ordinarily translated as "conceive" does not mean conception in the modern, technical sense of the term. The fertilization of an egg by a sperm is still in some respects mysterious to us today, even with the aid of modern technology, and the Hebrew language of 1000 BC did not have a word to describe fertilization as we know it now. This suggests caution in using Psalm 51 simplistically to identify a precise point in the procreative process at which human beings should be granted certain rights. Nevertheless, the language of Psalm 51:5 does communicate, in nonscientific terms, David's interest in the very beginnings of his existence in his mother's womb.

What do his words, inspired by the Holy Spirit, tell us about the earliest days of human life? First, the fact that he uses the first person pronoun, "me," is suggestive. Whatever this thing was in the earliest stages of growth in his mother's womb, he refers to it as *himself.* This indicates a continuity of identity with himself as the author of this psalm. Furthermore, it is quite significant that he refers to himself in his earliest days as someone implicated in sin. His language of being brought forth "in iniquity" and conceived "in sin" raises the question whether it is in fact he himself who is implicated or perhaps his parents who sinned in bringing him into existence. In the larger context of this psalm, David is intent on confessing *his own* sin, and thus his parents' sinfulness is irrelevant unless his own sinfulness is at issue as well. In fact, the idea that David was a sinner from his earliest days in the womb is perfectly consistent with Paul's later teaching in Romans 5:12–19, as reflected in the Christian doctrine of original sin. In the sin of one man, Adam, all have become sinners. David's sinful character, therefore, did not arise from his own voluntary actions sometime after birth, but was acquired through his association with the father of the human race. But if David confesses himself a sinner from his embryonic state, then as an embryo he possessed some sort of *moral accountability* (i.e., the ability to be held guilty of sin) and existed in a moral relationship with God. Both of these characteristics can be true only of an image bearer. David's words, then, implicitly communicate his apprehension of himself, even before birth, as an image-bearing human person.

Many writers have also cited Psalm 139 to make similar points. In this psalm David reflects upon the sovereign and all-knowing character of God's care for his people. The particularly relevant verses read:

> For you formed my inward parts;
>   you knitted me together in my mother's womb.
> I praise you, for I am fearfully and wonderfully made.
> Wonderful are your works;
>   my soul knows it very well.
> My frame was not hidden from you,
> when I was being made in secret,
>   intricately woven in the depths of the earth.
> Your eyes saw my unformed substance;
> in your book were written, every one of them,
>   the days that were formed for me,
>   when as yet there was none of them. (Ps. 139:13–16)

At least two points are worth noting. First, as in Psalm 51, the psalmist speaks of the developing fetus as himself, not as something other than him or as something that would become him. He uses first person pronouns, "me" and "my." This again suggests an intimate continuity between the being that lives outside of the womb and the being that developed in the womb. The fetus who developed into the psalmist was nothing other than David himself. Second, God's care for and interest in this fetus are striking. God of course knows every creature and cares for them all. But as Jesus explained, God does not show the same kind of care or personal involvement for every kind of creature: "Look at the birds of the air; they neither sow nor reap nor gather into barns, and yet your heavenly Father feeds them. Are you not of more value than they? . . . Consider the lilies of the field. . . . But if God so clothes the grass of the field, which today is alive and tomorrow is thrown into the oven, will he not much more clothe you, O you of little faith?" (Matt. 6:26–30). God has a special concern for his human creation, and it is precisely this sort of special concern that Psalm 139:13–16 describes. The providential care that God bestowed upon the unborn David is the kind that befits a human person, an image bearer of God, and not some lesser form of life.

Perhaps the biblical passage that has provoked the most discussion about the status of the unborn is Exodus 21:22–25: "When men strive together and hit a pregnant woman, so that her children come out, but there is no harm, the one who hit her shall surely be fined, as the woman's husband shall impose on him, and he shall pay as the judges determine. But if there is harm, then you shall pay life for life, eye for eye, tooth for tooth, hand for hand, foot for foot, burn for burn, wound for wound, stripe for stripe." This piece of Mosaic legislation is significant because the legal value that it places upon an unborn child reveals an underlying presupposition that unborn human life is worthy of protection similar to that of other human life. Granted, determining what the child's "coming out" and what "harm" refer to have been controversial. Many interpreters, defending a pro-life position, have argued that the first incident describes a premature birth, in which the child "comes out" earlier than normal but is not otherwise "harmed." This allegedly explains why only a fine is imposed, presumably to compensate for the pregnant woman's discomfort and distress. Many pro-life interpreters have then argued that the second incident refers to fetal death. In this case, there is "harm" in that the baby has died, which requires the imposition of the *lex talionis* penalty: life for life. The upshot of this interpretation is that the unborn child's life is valued just as highly as the life of one who is born, for murder requires the "life for life" penalty just as this extinction of fetal life does.

Other interpreters have offered a counterargument, which some writers have used to support a pro-choice position in which the fetus is not valued as an ordinary human person. According to this interpretation, the first scenario describes a miscarriage rather than a premature birth, and the loss of the fetus's life draws only a fine as its penalty. Furthermore, this interpretation takes the "harm" referred to in the second scenario as pertaining to the pregnant woman, not the fetus. Thus, only if the woman herself is injured or killed is the strict justice of the *lex talionis* to be applied.

Several considerations make the common pro-life interpretation more plausible than the common pro-choice interpretation. First, the word that is translated as "her children" is the ordinary Hebrew word for a child who is already born, and not the word that refers to a small fetus. Second, in Scripture the word that is translated as "come out" refers to a live birth and never to a miscarriage, except in a couple of cases when the child is specifically identified as dead. These facts, combined with the absence of the ordinary Hebrew word used to describe miscarriage, strongly suggest that the first scenario described in the text is not a miscarriage but a premature birth, and hence that the "harm" which is present in the second scenario refers to the child and not the mother. Furthermore, Meredith G. Kline has argued that, even if the first scenario does describe a miscarriage, the unborn child is valued no less than a person who is already born. Kline's argument from the Hebrew text concludes that the penalty in the first scenario, which is to be "imposed" by the husband and "determined" by the judges, is substantially the same as the *lex talionis* penalty for the second scenario. Taking the *lex talionis* not as prescribing literal application but as a formula demanding strict, proportionate punishment, Kline argues that the way the punishment is described in the first scenario communicates exactly this same idea as the *lex talionis* (even up to the point of allowing death as the penalty for a death inflicted). Thus the "harm" that is done to either mother or child alike, under both scenarios, is to be recompensed by a proportionate penalty, whether corporally or through a fine.

Various scholars have made other arguments in order to demonstrate a high biblical view of the unborn child. For example, Scripture often speaks of miscarriage as a great curse and tragedy (e.g., Ex. 23:26; Hos. 9:14), a fact difficult to understand if prenatal life is not greatly prized. But the final biblical argument to be considered here is drawn from Luke 1:35, in which the angel Gabriel explains to Mary how she, though a virgin, would conceive and bear a son. Some writers have presented a general biblical argument based upon the incarnation of the Lord Jesus Christ, resting their case on the fact that the Son became incarnate *from conception*, and that he proceeded through all of the stages of human life, from the womb through adulthood and unto death. Instead of coming into this world in the humanity of a full-grown adult, Christ redeemed us by experiencing all the steps of the life of a human person. If stated simplistically, this argument provokes serious objections. Given the doctrine that the incarnate Lord Jesus pre-existed as the second person of the Godhead, his personhood did not begin with his conception and thus his experience of embryonic personhood does not tell us anything about whether other people become persons at the time of fertilization.

Whatever the weaknesses of some versions of this argument, I believe that the words of Luke 1:35 do in fact lend support to a high view of human embryonic life. Gabriel says to Mary: "The Holy Spirit will come upon you, and the power of the Most High will overshadow you; therefore the child to be born will be called holy— the Son of God." It is crucial to recognize that this verse alludes to Exodus 40:34–35. The language of the original Greek text that describes the power of the Most High overshadowing Mary is also the language that the Septuagint (the Greek translation of the Old Testament) uses to describe the Shekinah glory cloud that overshadowed the newly completed tabernacle under the authority of Moses. This Shekinah glory cloud is frequently identified as a manifestation of the Holy Spirit himself in the Old Testament (e.g., Neh. 9:19–20; Isa. 63:11–14; Hag. 2:5) and is even identified with the Spirit of God who hovered over creation in Genesis 1:2 (as evident in the Hebrew text of Deut. 32:11). What is the significance of all of this? Gabriel's words in Luke 1:35 call our minds back not only to the Spirit's work in the re-creation act of constructing the tabernacle but even to his work in creation itself. The Spirit overshadowed the first creation, bringing forth human beings, created in his own image and likeness, as his climactic work. And here in Luke 1 the Spirit overshadows the new creation, working in Mary to bring forth a child, one who is "the *Son* of God," that is, one who bears the image and likeness of God. Luke 1:35, therefore, alerts us to the fact that the son of Mary is the second Adam, the true and consummate divine image bearer, a point that Paul made a cornerstone of his own theology (see Rom. 5:15–19 and 1 Cor. 15:22).

We should not miss the larger point. Mary has asked how she could have become pregnant, given her virginity (Luke 1:34). The answer to her question is that the Holy Spirit's action in making her pregnant is the very action that has produced one who is, in his *human* nature as the second Adam, the *image of God*. In other words, the embryonic Jesus was not a person simply because he was the eternal Son of God, but he was an image bearer of God in his humanity. If being an image bearer entails the highest possible created dignity, then the virgin conception of the Lord Jesus Christ indicates that the image of God exists even in embryonic human life, and thus that human life even from its earliest days is due the most profound respect.

We have observed a number of biblical considerations that confirm my earlier theological reflections on the image of God. Scripture and hence Christian theology impute dignity to human beings as God's image bearers and reckon this image-bearing dignity to extend back to the earliest days of human existence. Our considerations to this point, however, have not provided us with an *exact* time at which a human person originates. Even Psalm 51:5 and Luke 1:35, given the imprecision of the Hebrew word for "conceive" and the mystery surrounding Christ's incarnation, do not identify fertilization itself or another time shortly thereafter as *the* point of image-bearing origin. For the original readers of Scripture this lack of specificity may not have had any practical consequence. But today our detailed knowledge of fertilization and of the growth of the embryo from that point forward raises more precise questions. And the ethical questions that face us today, such as controversies over the "morning-after" pill and embryonic stem-cell research, mean that whether human life should be protected beginning at fertilization or at another point even a short time thereafter can make a big practical difference. Thus we need to explore whether we are able to make a more precise identification of when image-bearing human personhood begins, for purposes of guiding our ethical deliberation about significant issues such as abortion and embryonic research.

The Decisiveness of Fertilization

Our discussion here will take us beyond the exegesis of Scripture and perhaps even beyond *theological* reasoning, strictly speaking. Many questions that modern technology has put to us—due to our scientific knowledge of early human existence and our ability to research, to manipulate, and to destroy embryonic life—have no ready biblical and theological answer. But the scientific knowledge that we have attained provides us with crucial pieces of information that do allow us to make the necessary urgent moral judgments. In other words, the fact that modern science forces us to ask novel ethical questions means that we must turn right back to modern science to determine precisely what happens in the early weeks after fertilization. Scientific facts themselves cannot answer ethical questions. But our ability to answer many ethical questions depends upon our perception and identification of the particular circumstances that prompt the questions in the first place. Thus the question before us is this: given the biblical conviction that image-bearing human life extends back into the womb and even to the earliest days of existence, does modern science provide us with information about those earliest days of existence that permits us to conclude whether fertilization or some other point shortly thereafter is the beginning point of human personhood? I am not a trained scientist. But given the knowledge that scientifically trained people can provide the rest of us, I conclude that identifying fertilization as this beginning point is the most compelling conclusion.

The argument, in summary, is that fertilization is a unique and radical event. Before fertilization there is nothing recognizably identifiable as the human life that will develop into a full-grown human person. After fertilization, the embryo experiences an unbroken and continuous development, and at no point in that development does the embryo/fetus/child undergo a radical transformation from one sort of being into another sort.

What happens at fertilization that marks such a radical transformation, the likes of which occurs at no other time in subsequent human development? Fertilization is a process of about twenty-four hours during which a sperm penetrates an egg. The egg's cytoplasm and the sperm's nuclear contents merge (called "syngamy") and form a set of forty-six chromosomes. What is crucial to note is that this newly formed zygote is clearly *not* the same entity as either the sperm or egg prior to fertilization. Both the sperm and the egg are genetically different from the zygote, even though the genetic material that each contains contributes to the zygote's genetic makeup. Neither the sperm nor the egg has any inherent ability, under any circumstances, to develop into a mature human being. Sperm and egg are living things, but they are not designed for independent life, and they die quickly if they do not experience fertilization. When fertilization does occur, however, a new, genetically unique being comes into existence that is indeed designed for independent life. From a scientific perspective, fertilization effects a radical transformation in which two entities, genetically different from each other and unable to survive without each other, combine in order to form a genetically unique living human entity that is capable of developing into a full-grown human being.

The following question then arises: is there any other point in the subsequent development of this newly fertilized embryo at which another radical transformation takes place? Writers have proposed a number of different stages in that development as the point at which personhood begins, but a fair analysis demonstrates that none of them constitute a radical transformation from one kind of being into another kind. We can examine some of those proposed stages and reflect upon why looking to any of them as a decisive transformative point is arbitrary and unjustified.

Most easy to refute are proposals that point to stages that come relatively late in the process of development. Two such stages, in reverse chronological order, are *birth* and *viability*. In contemporary Western culture there is widespread condemnation and abhorrence of infanticide, though a few radical writers have defended it. Could *birth*, however, be a point of decisive transformation from one sort of being into another sort, such that personhood and thus a right to life might begin there? There may be an initial plausibility in this suggestion, since at birth a living being ceases to exist in another person's body and no longer depends fully upon it for sustenance. At birth this being begins to breathe on its own, takes in nourishment through its mouth, and becomes capable of existence independent of its mother. Though birth is a decisive event in a human life, however, it is clearly not a radical transformation in the kind of being that it is. Circumstances change significantly at birth, but the baby herself does not. The lungs and mouth that begin to take in air and nourishment after birth were fully capable of doing such things a day before birth. The day on which her mother happened to go into labor had no effect on the baby's inherent ability to live independently of her mother. Thus, birth does not constitute a shift in the nature of a human being.

What about *viability*? Some writers agree that the somewhat arbitrary date of birth does not mark a decisive change in the nature of the baby but have suggested that the ability to live outside of the womb does. American jurisprudence since *Roe vs. Wade* depends significantly on this idea. But attributing personhood and human rights to babies at the point at which they become viable for life outside the womb also has serious difficulties. Chief among these difficulties is that it is impossible to identify a certain point in fetal development at which viability is attained. With the advance of medical technology, the point at which a fetus might be considered viable is much earlier today than it was a hundred years ago, and most likely it will be earlier one hundred years from now than it is today. Focusing on the present day, we must conclude that a fetus developing in a mother who lives in a first-world country becomes viable long before a fetus developing in a mother who lives in a third-world country. In fact, the very same fetus may be viable in the morning, when his mother wakes up in Miami, and nonviable in the evening, after his mother has traveled to a remote village in Haiti. The fact is, no point of radical transformation occurs in developing fetuses at which they turn from being nonviable to being viable. Thus assigning a certain fetal age as that of "viability" and making that the point at which we ascribe personhood and human rights to fetuses is arbitrary.

If birth and viability are dismissed as decisive points for determining human personhood, what about earlier stages in fetal development? Two such candidates are the point of "quickening" and the point at which the nervous system is fully integrated. Some considerations drawn from Christian theology do lend some plausible support for these candidates, but these too must ultimately be rejected.

Many Christian theologians of an earlier age viewed "quickening," or "animation," as a crucial point in the development of the unborn child, and not without reason. According to Christian theology, the human person as image bearer of God is not a body alone but body *and* soul. Quickening, or the point at which a mother can first feel the baby moving within her, was often deemed to be the point of ensoulment, that is, when God creates a living soul in the developing human body. According to this reasoning, quickening marks the beginning of truly *human* life. There are difficulties with this view from both the physical and the spiritual angles, however. From the physical angle, modern scientific knowledge of fetal development recognizes no decisive change in the fetus that causes the mother to feel her child for the first time. From the spiritual angle, as noted in chapter 5, Scripture does not inform us how or at precisely what point the soul comes into existence. To identify it as happening at the moment of quickening, especially when no decisive physical change in the fetus is discernable, is arbitrary, and thus quickening is a poor candidate for the point at which human rights begin.

Looking to the time when the fetus's nervous system is fully integrated (around the twentieth week) also is a decision that is attractive given certain historic Christian notions. Some streams of the Christian tradition have defined a human person as an individual substance of a rational nature, a view that still finds currency among some contemporary Roman Catholics. If rationality is required for human personhood, some have argued, then a fetus must have the physical apparatus capable of rational activity, and it does not attain this until the integration of its nervous system. This argument fails for several reasons. For one thing, the argument relies on a definition of human personhood that overemphasizes rationality. Earlier I acknowledged that rationality is an aspect of the image of God. But I also argued that the image of God has many aspects, and the absence of one or another of these aspects does not result in the absence of the image itself. To identify a certain point in fetal development when the fetus attains rationality as the point when it attains personhood and/or the image of God is therefore an unjustified move. Furthermore, is it really convincing that the fetus becomes a rational being at the point of integration of the nervous system? Even if scientists could identify a discrete moment when the nervous system becomes fully integrated, the fetus hardly begins to think or to act in what we ordinarily think of as a rational way. The fetus may have gained something necessary for rational behavior—a fully integrated nervous system—but such activity is still only potential, requiring further development. Yet this same fetus in the days before integration of the nervous system also had potential for rational behavior, just at a less developed stage. Thus, integration of the nervous system fails to constitute a decisive transformation of a fetus from one sort of being into another sort.

All of the stages discussed thus far are qualitatively different from fertilization, considered simply in a scientific sense. At none of these stages does a radical transformation occur in the kind of being that exists. This concurs with what we would have expected to find in light of the biblical and theological teaching discussed earlier. Scripture compels us to the conclusion that a human being, from the very earliest days of its existence, is an image bearer of God and thus due all of the respect and protection that such a status entails. These stages do not take us back to these earliest days, and thus the fact that we find no radical transformation from one kind of being into another kind is perfectly harmonious with biblical teaching. But there is at least one additional stage that does take us back very early in human development. This stage may be identified as "individuation," that is, the point at which an *individual* human being comes to exist. According to some advocates of this argument, the embryo is a living human entity beginning at fertilization, but it is not an individual human life until about three weeks later. Only when this individual human being comes into existence do we have an entity that could conceivably be recognized as a human person who possesses a full right to life.

In my judgment this is by far the strongest counterargument to the claim that bearing the image of God begins at fertilization. It seems reasonable to grant that where there is no individual there is no person or image bearer. It is also true that there are serious arguments in support of the claim that no individual human being exists before the end of the third week after fertilization. If this position is embraced, furthermore, it would still constitute a significant challenge to the reigning pro-choice orthodoxy, even if it would open the door to the morality of using the morning-after pill and pursuing embryonic stem-cell research. Nevertheless I believe that this position should also be rejected.

Why have writers argued that no individual human being exists prior to three weeks after fertilization? First, some of them have appealed to certain aspects of embryonic life during the first several days of existence that involve *gaining* individuality rather than possessing it from the start. For example, during the initial seventy-two hours or so of embryonic life, messenger RNA (mRNA) from the mother plays a role in directing embryonic development, until embryonic genes take full control. This is not decisive proof of lack of individuality, however. The presence of outside influence upon development is hardly incompatible with distinct individual existence and, as other writers have argued, the embryo is still the primary organizer of its growing process even during these opening days. Another alleged piece of evidence that the newly formed embryo lacks individuality is the fact that until the blastocyst stage (four to six days after fertilization), each of the embryonic cells is undifferentiated and possesses totipotency. In other words, each of the cells has the potential to develop into any particular kind of human cell. But again this fails to prove lack of individuality. It is true that the parts, viewed in abstraction from the embryo as a whole, could develop in any number of different directions. But the parts do not operate except in coordination with the whole. The embryo has not yet decided, so to speak, which parts will develop in which directions, but the way in which each part does develop is explicable only in light of the purposeful growth of the integrated embryonic life.

The most serious and challenging argument for lack of individuality during the first three weeks after fertilization is drawn from the phenomenon of twinning. During this initial period in an embryo's life, the single embryo may form into twins, resulting in *two* embryos of identical genetic makeup. Furthermore, in even rarer cases the twin embryos recombine so that again a single embryo alone continues to develop. The argument latent in this data is not difficult to discover. If an early embryo might turn into two embryos and then back into one, then it cannot be until after this possibility has disappeared that we have an *individual*.

I suggest two responses to this argument. First, the great majority of embryos do not twin (or recombine). Most embryos thus experience a continuous line of development during their first three weeks and on into the weeks that follow. The argument just presented, therefore, proposes that a developing embryo's individuality begins at a point at which nothing decisive actually occurs in the great majority of cases. The fact that *some* embryos twin during the first three weeks does not mean that *all* of them are not individuals during this period. This prompts my second response. Why some embryos twin and why some of these recombine is still largely a mystery that science has not explained. It is a mystery whether something genetically inherent in the particular embryo drives it to twin (and maybe recombine) or whether a force outside of the embryo causes this phenomenon. If the former is true, most embryos have no potential to twin, which directly undercuts the lack-of-individuality argument. Another mystery is the precise relationship of the single embryo to the twin embryos that emerge from it. Is one of the twins the continuing original embryo and the other twin a new being? If so, there is no reason to conclude that an individual human being did not exist before twinning. And when recombination occurs, do the embryos literally *recombine* or is the newly single embryo the same being as one of the twins (which would mean that the other twin has died)? If the latter is the case, then again there is no need to deny individuality during the first three weeks even to those embryos that twin and recombine.

As conceded above, the twinning phenomenon is the aspect of early fetal development that raises the most serious objections to the claim that image-bearing human existence begins at fertilization. Nevertheless, given the current state of scientific knowledge about twinning, this phenomenon fails to prove lack of individuality during the first three weeks. The final conclusion, therefore, is that modern scientific learning shows fertilization to be a *unique* event in which *a new kind of living being comes into existence*. If Scripture compels us to conclude that human beings are image bearers of God from their earliest days, and if science asks us when exactly that identity is established, the evidence that science provides suggests that the answer to that question must be fertilization.

Implications: Abortion and Embryonic Stem-Cell Research

We can conclude that a human embryo, even from the point of fertilization, is an image bearer of God and worthy of all due respect. But this is not merely a question of theoretical interest but one of great practical relevance. I have already drawn important conclusions about contraception and assisted reproduction from the conviction that embryonic human life should be protected. Given this conviction, the basic Christian stance in regard to abortion and embryonic stem-cell research is rather plain. But in light of the significance of these two issues in contemporary life, we should briefly examine them.

Some discussion of abortion is particularly appropriate since most Christians at some point in their lives find themselves or their wives pregnant, and many face unplanned pregnancies or pregnancies that pose unexpected hardships. It is often much easier to take a pro-life stance in theory than it is to live consistently with the theory. Situations that make abortion a temptation are not merely trials for the expectant mothers (and fathers), however, but trials for the church at large. These situations beckon the church to respond with the love that ought to characterize it and to set it apart from the world. Some Christians become pregnant out of wedlock, and in such cases the church ought to be eager to forgive and restore the sinner who repents, in order to avoid driving such people to abortion out of a sense of shame or a hope to conceal their sins. Some Christians become pregnant through rape, and the church ought to show abundant compassion to such women who have suffered a horrible and violent crime, and who may be inclined to abort in order to wipe away a constant reminder of a terrifying event. Other Christians face pregnancy in the face of overwhelming financial hardship or with the prospect of bearing severely handicapped children who will be unable to enjoy a normal life and whose care will place a heavy burden on the parents. In all such circumstances the church's obligation is to exhibit the kind of merciful and self-sacrificing love that Christ showed to her.

Christians who show such love to one another, not merely in word but also in action, exhibit a true pro-life ethic. When they uphold their sisters and brothers experiencing burdensome pregnancies and pledge their time and resources to contribute to the care that these children will require, they bestow profound assistance to those who might otherwise succumb to the pressures to abort that society often imposes. Here, in the Christlike love of the church, we find perhaps the best answer to the question whether abortion is permissible in certain extreme cases, such as rape or a severely handicapped fetus. Rather than compounding evils by taking the life of an innocent image bearer, how much better for the members of the church to share each other's burdens. Christians are called to suffer in this life, yet suffering with one another not only lightens each other's loads but also offers a beautiful witness to what has been called our "culture of death."

The rare pregnancy that threatens the mother's life is one case that is not so obviously addressed by this moral exhortation. In my judgment, abortion is justified in such circumstances through the general principle that people may defend their own lives and the lives of others from those who would take them unjustly. Of course the baby who threatens his mother's life cannot be regarded as guilty of a crime, but in ordinary life people may justly defend even against those who threaten another's life without guilty intent. Such an occurrence is still a profound tragedy, and here too the church is compelled to exhibit love to those who find themselves is such a terrible situation.

The issue of embryonic stem-cell research is less relevant to the concerns of this book, since it is not a moral question that faces most Christians in the midst of their everyday lives. But it is a question that faces some Christians engaged in scientific research, and the hoped-for benefits of such research promise to aid many Christians who suffer. Most immediately, it is a pressing and controversial public policy issue that prompts ordinary Christians to wonder about their own stance. While we are not focused upon public policy questions, some guidance on embryonic stem-cell research can aid Christians as they form their own views on this controversy.

Stem-cell research receives so much attention for the simple reason that discovering how stem cells work and how they might be manipulated holds tremendous prospects for treating a range of illnesses and disabilities. Stem cells are distinct from other human cells in that they are not fully differentiated. In other words, they are not already serving as a certain type of human cell but, as undifferentiated or at least not fully differentiated, they are able to develop into human cells of a variety of types. There are different kinds of stem cells. The most valuable to medical researchers are "pluripotent," which are undifferentiated and are capable of developing into any kind of tissue in the human body. Other stem cells are "multipotent," which can form into some but not all kinds of human tissue, and "unipotent," which can form into one kind only. These latter sorts of stem cells are more differentiated and thus less valuable to researchers, because their potential uses are more restricted. The moral rub is that human embryos (unlike adult human beings) are a rich source of pluripotent stem cells, and hence interest has surged in creating embryos in order to experiment on their stem cells, or least in using embryos that have been created for other reasons but will be discarded otherwise.

Arguing against stem-cell research can be difficult, because many people have raised such high expectations for the results of such research. We are told that cures for so many diseases and the alleviation of so much suffering are just around the corner. To argue for the protection of a newly fertilized embryo when millions of already existing and suffering individuals might be helped requires courage. Nevertheless, if embryos are indeed image bearers of God beginning at fertilization, then this conclusion is necessary. Throughout history people have proffered ingenious arguments for harming some human beings (usually those deemed weak, insignificant, and dispensable) for the benefit of the many, and the present stem-cell controversy presents a similar scenario in different garb. Destroying the life of the weak and insignificant who may have no voice of their own is too high a price to pay to relieve the suffering of the many (who are often well-funded and vocal). Christians are called to suffer in this life in union with their suffering Lord and are called to a Christlike, self-sacrificial love. Even if they could be certain that stem-cell research would lead to cures for their ailments, Christians should be willing to forgo their own healing for the sake of defending vulnerable human beings.

Several other considerations based on general moral principle bolster this conclusion. One consideration is that many of the touted benefits of stem-cell research are entirely speculative at this point. The beneficial results are easy to imagine, and it is plausible to think that they are attainable. But researchers and their advocates have made plenty of big promises in the past that never materialized. Experimenting on and destroying image bearers, and spending billions of dollars in the process, are all the more hard to justify given the uncertainty of the evidence that the benefits will be realized. Another consideration is that embryos are not the only source of stem cells that may prove beneficial for medical research. Umbilical cord blood, for example, is a fertile and rather plentiful source of stem cells that has already been put to good medical use (for example, umbilical cord blood stem cells can be used in place of donated adult bone marrow for bone marrow transplants, with better results under certain circumstances). Perhaps even more significantly, scientists have recently developed methods of attaining pluripotent stem cells without destroying embryos in the process. These developments may make embryonic stem-cell research unnecessary altogether.

Conclusion

Many beginning-of-life bioethical issues depend upon a proper view of the origin of individual human life, and we have seen that Scripture teaches Christians to view embryos as image bearers of God even in their earliest days. Given what we now know about fertilization and the development of young human life through pregnancy, the evidence drives us to the conclusion that respect for image-bearing human life should extend all the way back to fertilization. The implications of this conviction have become profound in our own day. Christians can maintain such a view only by resisting great pressure from the world and sometimes even from their own sinful temptations in the face of suffering. Thus, here is a rich occasion for Christians to exhibit the courage that Christian faith produces and to love and to uphold one another with the love of Christ so that our faltering courage does not fail.

PART 3

THE END OF LIFE

"The years of our life are seventy, or even by reason of strength eighty; yet their span is but toil and trouble; they are soon gone, and we fly away. . . . So teach us to number our days that we may get a heart of wisdom" (Ps. 90:10, 12). Reflecting upon the brevity and difficulties of life is not an attractive activity. But Scripture exhorts us to take time to step back from the distractions of everyday life and to consider our lives as a whole. Despite the joys and opportunities that many people experience, Psalm 90 reminds us that earthly life is short and hard, and will one day end. That is somewhat depressing, perhaps, but the psalmist informs us that taking stock of life and death in this way will give us a heart of wisdom.

We now turn to death, dying, and preparation for those inevitable events. The experience of death and dying is a constant of all human history, and thus many of the moral issues that it provokes are perennial. But the explosion of biomedical technology in recent generations has altered the landscape at the end of life in countless ways. Many previously untreatable diseases are now curable, the lives of many terminally ill patients can be significantly prolonged, and the pain produced by fatal diseases can be minimized. One significant side effect of these medical advancements is that far fewer people today die at home, in familiar surroundings with family by their side, and far more people die in hospitals or in other institutional settings. Both *how* people die and *where* people die, therefore, look much different from the ways of generations past. Yet the fact *that* people continue to die means, for all of the differences, that the same basic human and moral predicament that faced every preceding generation still faces every person today.

These next three chapters examine death and dying both as a universal human predicament and as a new challenge in the light of recent technological and social developments. Following the plan of this book, I approach these issues in the context of the broader Christian moral life. Like all human beings, Christians must die, but Scripture calls us to die "in Christ," and the death that we die cannot be separated from the life that we have lived throughout our earthly pilgrimage. The better a person embraces the doctrines and virtues of the Christian faith through all of life, the better that person is prepared to die.

7

APPROACHING DEATH: DYING AS A WAY OF LIFE

What is the proper Christian attitude toward death? What responsibility do Christians have to live their whole lives in preparation for death? In order to answer these questions, we should investigate how to cultivate the proper virtues and how to give careful thought to practical issues such as financial responsibility and living wills. Then we will consider organ donation in light of these broader questions about preparing for death. These discussions will enable us to explore important questions about accepting and refusing medical treatment—both for oneself and on behalf of others.

The Christian's Attitude toward Death
Before investigating the practical ways in which Christians should prepare to die, we do well to ponder the general attitude that they should adopt toward death. Is death an enemy, a natural inevitability, or perhaps a friend? As explored in chapter 2, Scripture presents clear answers about such questions. But Christians hear not only the voice of Scripture but also the voice of the broader, unbelieving world. This latter voice communicates in both obvious and subtle ways—through television, film, books, and the opinions of medical professionals from whom the news of death often comes. Christians often find it difficult

to disentangle themselves from the perspectives on death that they imbibe from the surrounding culture, and thus we must be alert to the ways in which the world views death.

Predominant views about death have shifted significantly in America over the past several generations. A few landmark books, none of them written from a Christian perspective, illustrate this shift. The first is the 1949 memoir by John Gunther, *Death Be Not Proud*. This moving and memorable book is a father's account of his seventeen-year-old son's battle with a brain tumor that eventually took his life. The story is fascinating in several respects. Gunther's son, an intelligent and talented boy headed for Harvard, is admirable in many ways, both in his attitude in the face of severe setbacks and in the courage he demonstrated in submitting to terrible treatments. Furthermore, the Gunther family had access to many prominent physicians and was able to secure a number of cutting-edge and experimental procedures for their son, thereby raising profound ethical questions about whether death should be fought at any cost, physical or financial. But the Gunthers, by their own admission, experienced little moral doubt about such things and pursued every route that held out the slightest chance of recovery. Death, for the Gunthers, was clearly an enemy, to be fought with every available resource. Most fascinating of all, perhaps, is the fact that young Johnny Gunther, as far as his father was aware, never knew that he was going to die. Neither his parents nor doctors informed him that all possible medical procedures had failed. The author admits to lying to his son during times of setback, hiding bad news from him and instead giving him reason for optimism. They did not want to break his spirit. Thus death overtook Johnny Gunther unawares, though his physicians and parents knew that death was inevitable.

This idea of death as a great enemy—to be fought, repressed, and denied wherever possible—has come under critical scrutiny in subsequent generations in America. One significant figure who articulated a different perspective was Elisabeth Kübler-Ross, a Swiss physician who penned the influential book *On Death and Dying* in 1969. Kübler-Ross looked upon a world in which people avoided talking about death, particularly with dying people. She lamented the repression and denial provoked by modern anxieties about death and suggested that we can attain inner peace if we face and accept the reality of our own death. What we tend to repress in our unconscious mind through various defense mechanisms must be brought to conscious awareness. Based upon her extensive clinical work with the dying, Kübler-Ross identified a series of stages that most people experience after learning that they have a terminal illness: denial, anger, bargaining, depression, and finally acceptance. Family and caregivers, she argued, ought to help patients to work through these stages, encouraging them to express their thoughts and feelings along the way. Provided that there is enough time between the diagnosis of terminal illness and death, the patient who works through these stages can attain a state of acceptance and even peace (if not happiness). Kübler-Ross observed that hope of medical recovery tends to persist through all of these stages. When death finally comes, she explained, we should allow loved ones to go through their own experience of anger and despair and to express their feelings. Speaking to them of the love of God in such situations is cruel and inappropriate.

Many of Kübler-Ross's ideas have gained influence in subsequent years through the hospice movement and popular books about dying. Sherwin B. Nuland's *How We Die: Reflections on Life's Final Chapter*, for instance, sets out to "demythologize" the process of dying. By explaining biologically and clinically what happens when people die, Nuland hoped to relieve people of many of their fears of dying and of the self-deception and disillusionment created by anxiety about the unknown. Another example is *Dying Well: Peace and Possibilities at the End of Life*, by physician and hospice director Ira Byock. According to Byock, American society is unfamiliar with death. Thus it tends to isolate loved ones who are dying and to miss opportunities to foster human relationships at the end of life. He proposed that the end of life actually holds great possibilities for strengthening bonds among people, for creating moments of deep human significance, and for growing morally as human beings. Byock hence sought to foster these experiences at the end of life and advocated discussion of spiritual matters.

Directly or indirectly, the Christian who lives in American culture has been exposed to various theories and practices of death and dying. In light of the biblical theology of death examined in chapter 2, Christians should probably look upon these various sentiments with both appreciation and sadness. When they read Gunther's memoir, they can surely appreciate the horror and hopelessness that death evokes without Christ, for death is indeed an enemy and a source of despair apart from the gospel. Yet Christians can hardly countenance the elaborate scheme to hide the full seriousness of medical problems and the immanence of death from a young man, such that death would take him by surprise. While no one would wish to strip someone of the desire to fight for life when that is still medically possible, Christians recognize that death is far too serious a matter to justify deceiving someone about the fact that he must face it soon. In light of this, Christians can find many things attractive about the new perspective cultivated by Kübler-Ross. Acknowledging the reality of death and confronting the challenges of dying seems much more in line with Christian conviction about the seriousness of death and the need to love the dying person. Certainly many Christians have profited from open conversations made possible by revised attitudes about death and by resources such as hospice. Nevertheless, some of the ideas inculcated by this newer perspective on dying are unsatisfactory from a biblical standpoint. Death is not merely something natural, the latter stage in the larger process of life. Death, in the ultimate sense, is unnatural, not a part of the world as God designed it. If death is a curse and brings people before the judgment of God, then they surely cannot attain true peace about death simply by expressing their feelings about it. If death is the diametric opposite of what God's image bearers were created to experience (namely, life), then dying with genuine dignity is hard to imagine, no matter how much love friends and family show to a dying person.

The meaning and experience of death has been transformed for the Christian. Christians need no longer be trapped in the sort of dilemmas about death that haunt the broader culture. In the broader culture people tend either to recognize the horror of death and therefore to avoid confronting it or to encourage open acknowledgment and discussion of death but to reconceive it as something natural and acceptable. For the Christian, death remains an enemy that produces sorrow and grief among the dying and their loved ones, yet by virtue of Christ's work of redemption death has been defeated. Christians may genuinely look forward to being with Christ in glory when they die and to being raised up on the last day with glorified bodies.

Both in its horror and in its hope, death remains an event of utmost gravity for the Christian. How then should Christians prepare for this inevitable experience? How should they undertake the Christian life even in times of youth and health, when death seems far off, so that they are not caught surprised and unprepared for death when it comes? We can consider both the perennial questions about death as a human experience and the new challenges introduced by contemporary medical technology and the institutionalization of death.

Death as Life-Defining

In the later Middle Ages and through the first centuries after the Reformation, both Protestant and Roman Catholic writers produced literature on the *ars moriendi*, the art of dying. Recognizing that death is an event of great weight and everlasting consequence, these writers taught that dying well does not come naturally but is a practice that must be learned. Furthermore, they saw dying as a practice that must be learned through the whole of life if it is to be executed well. Though writers from different churches described the *ars moriendi* in various ways, reflecting their different theological convictions, the general concern for preparing people to die was one that many professing Christians shared for many centuries, and for good reason.

Many people today express the sentiment that the best death is a sudden death that involves no extended period of pain or suffering. While such a perspective is eminently understandable, we should appreciate why so many people in other times and places regarded a sudden and unexpected death as a great misfortune. A sudden and unexpected death leaves no time to put one's house in order, no time to say goodbye to loved ones, no time to reconcile with those who are estranged, and, most importantly, no time to be sure that one is right with God. A death that is expected and gradual leaves time for preparation and wrapping up unfinished business. Some people still remind us of these things. Randy Pausch, for example, the forty-seven-year-old professor with terminal pancreatic cancer whose *The Last Lecture* is a best seller at the time I write this chapter, expresses his gratitude for the few months' notice that he had, which allowed him to give his last lecture at Carnegie Mellon University and to spend precious time with his family.

Yet sudden death often occurs, whether from natural or unnatural causes. The fact that we go through life not knowing the day of death, not knowing whether it will come tomorrow, though we feel well today, ought to give us pause. The only way truly to be prepared for this momentous event of death *is to be ready at all times*. If we make the effort to prepare in youth, in early adulthood, in middle age, or wherever we find ourselves in life's pilgrimage, we will not be left unprepared even if death comes tomorrow completely unexpectedly. The responsible Christian life involves having one's house in order *now*, cultivating relationships with loved ones *now*, reconciling with those who are estranged *now*, and taking account of one's standing before God *now*. If they are committed to these practices, Christians will be prepared for death—whether it is sudden or gradual—in a way that they would not otherwise be.

The words of Psalm 90 quoted at the outset of Part 3 counsel us "to number our days that we may get a heart of wisdom." Indeed, numbering our days involves gaining wisdom as well as a range of other virtues. Cultivating Christian virtues can prepare us for death, and hence help us to avoid the way of foolishness.

Faith

As considered in chapter 3, the virtue of faith is the fount of the other virtues. But faith should not be viewed as a means to an end, that is, as simply a means for attaining the other virtues. Rather, in the context of death the most important thing about faith is that it secures our right standing before God and therefore gives us confidence before him on the last day. Death is such a momentous event first and foremost because it ushers us into the presence of the living God before whom all must stand. By faith we are justified, declared righteous before God's throne of judgment (Rom. 3:23–26). By faith, therefore, we may be confident that death will bring us into the gracious presence of God rather than confront us with his wrath (Rom. 5:9). Faith in the Lord Jesus Christ, as proclaimed in the gospel, means that we need not go to our death anxious and afraid, wondering whether we will be saved or lost. Instead, by faith we approach death with gratitude and assurance of salvation. Becoming right with God is thus not something that can be delayed. Preparation for death, even when it seems far away, first of all requires us to reckon with our everlasting destiny. As Paul wrote to the Corinthian church, "We implore you on behalf of Christ, be reconciled to God. . . . Behold, now is the favorable time; behold, now is the day of salvation" (2 Cor. 5:20; 6:2).

We must remember, however, that faith is not a one-time act. It is not as though a person comes to Christ in faith at the very beginning of the Christian life and then moves on to other things. On the contrary, faith is to be the constant and abiding response of the Christian to God's grace through all of life. Faith is the means by which we are justified and is the fount of virtues not simply as a past act but as an ongoing trust in Christ. How is faith cultivated throughout life? Meditating upon Christ and his work is a task for every day and an encouragement for our faith, but God has ordained a special place for *the preaching of the Word of God* for evoking and nourishing faith in his people. In Romans 10:17 Paul explains: "Faith comes from hearing, and hearing through the word of Christ." Reading the Scriptures privately and as families can certainly be of great encouragement for our faith, but Paul identifies *hearing* the word *preached* as of particular importance for building faith. As he writes a few verses earlier, "How then will they call on him in whom they have not believed? And how are they to believe in him of whom they have never heard? And how are they to hear without someone preaching?" (Rom. 10:14).

There is probably nothing that better prepares people for death than being/becoming members of a faithful church of Jesus Christ where the Word that produces faith is proclaimed Sunday after Sunday. God also ordained sacraments—baptism and the Lord's Supper—to be administered alongside preaching. Sacraments are God's visible and tangible ways of setting Christ and his redeeming work before our sight, taste, and touch. Baptism symbolizes our dying with Christ and being resurrected with him (see Rom. 6:3–5)—not a bad preparation for our own death! In the Lord's Supper we are nourished by communing with the body and blood of Christ (1 Cor. 10:16). Partaking of the Supper is such a weighty thing that Paul calls us to examine ourselves each time we come to the table (1 Cor. 11:28). Thus we not only receive grace for building up our faith by partaking of the Supper but are also required to take account of ourselves and to stir up our faith when we are invited to eat and drink. In short, there is no more fundamental way to prepare for death than to grow in faith, and there is no better way to grow in faith than to hear the Word proclaimed weekly, to recall the grace of our baptism, and to participate in the Lord's Supper frequently.

Hope

Chapter 3 argued that hope is in some sense the first fruit of faith. Christian hope is not the "hope" of everyday speech that sets its sights on earthly things that are merely possible. Rather, Christian hope, founded in faith, looks ahead to Christ's second coming and the resurrection of our bodies, awaiting them not as possible but as certain and assured. Hope is crucial to cultivate as we prepare for death. Scripture trains us for the end of life by instilling in us a heavenly-minded, eschatological perspective that is the essence of hope.

Instead of cultivating a heavenly-minded hope, sinful human beings tend to be focused on the present things of this earth and are thus unprepared for death. The words of James 4:13–15 are sobering: "Come now, you who say, 'Today or tomorrow we will go into such and such a town and spend a year there and trade and make a profit'—yet you do not know what tomorrow will bring. What is your life? For you are a mist that appears for a little time and then vanishes. Instead you ought to say, 'If the Lord wills, we will live and do this or that.'" James confronts a problem endemic to human behavior in this world: conducting ourselves and making plans for the future without recognizing the tenuousness, precariousness, and brevity of life. Jesus spoke words similar to James's, calling the person who gives no thought to the end of life a fool. "And he told them a parable, saying, 'The land of a rich man produced plentifully, and he thought to himself, "What shall I do, for I have nowhere to store my crops?" And he said, "I will do this: I will tear down my barns and build larger ones, and there I will store all my grain and my goods. And I will say to my soul, Soul, you have ample goods laid up for many years; relax, eat, drink, be merry." But God said to him, "Fool! This night your soul is required of you, and the things you have prepared, whose will they be?"'" (Luke 12:16–20). Who of us has not acted like this fool, laying plans for the future without a thought to the fact that it may not be God's will that we live to execute them? How do we remedy this sinful tendency? What virtue should we cultivate for this purpose?

There is surely no better remedy to this sinful tendency than heavenly-mindedness, that abiding awareness of where our true home is even now and a genuine longing to enter that place with soul and body. Thus we must seek to grow in hope, that virtue which orients us with confidence toward the age to come. Paul probably had in mind people like the fool condemned by James and Jesus when he described "enemies of the cross of Christ. Their end is destruction, their god is their belly, and they glory in their shame, with minds set on earthly things" (Phil. 3:18–19). With minds on earthly things, they had no time to consider the brevity of life, but lived instead for their own worldly accomplishment and self-indulgence. Diametrically opposed to this way of life is that of the Christian described by Paul in the next verses: "But our citizenship is in heaven, and from it we await a Savior, the Lord Jesus Christ, who will transform our lowly body to be like his glorious body, by the power that enables him even to subject all things to himself" (Phil. 3:20–21). Heavenly-mindedness ought to crowd out earthly obsession in the believer. It ought to create hope in the imminent return of Christ to raise up our mortal bodies but also ought to make us conform our lives at present to the heavenly way of life. Paul's original readers knew what it was to be a citizen of one city while living far away from it. Philippi was a Roman colony and thus governed as a Roman city, and its citizens were reckoned as Roman citizens. As the residents of Philippi conducted themselves day by day as if they lived in Rome, so Paul called the Philippian Christians to conduct themselves day by day as though they belonged to heaven.

Paul presented similar themes in Colossians 3:1–4. Here again he appeals to his readers' hope in the return of Christ and exhorts them to make that hope determinative for their conduct in the present: "If then you have been raised with Christ, seek the things that are above, where Christ is, seated at the right hand of God. Set your minds on things that are above, not on things that are on earth. For you have died, and your life is hidden with Christ in God. When Christ, who is your life appears, then you also will appear with him in glory." Contrary to expectation, heavenly-mindedness is apparently the most practical thing imaginable, for in the rest of the chapter Paul explains a great number of concrete moral obligations that follow from this other-worldly orientation. The person who sets her mind on heaven, where the resurrected Christ already reigns and where we will join him in glory one day soon, will not be vulnerable to the trap of earthly obsessions. Death will not catch such a person unawares.

Christ's words in the Sermon on the Mount reinforce this point: "Blessed are those who hunger and thirst for righteousness, for they shall be satisfied" (Matt. 5:6). According to Paul in Philippians 3, those who have their minds set on earthly things focus upon their bellies, that is, their physical appetites. Hence they make plans about doing business and building barns that aim to satisfy physical needs and desires. But citizens of the kingdom of heaven, Jesus explains, are characterized by a different kind of hunger and thirst—for righteousness—and Jesus promises them satisfaction. Since Scripture makes clear that sin will always cling to us on earth, this promised satisfaction can be attained only in the age to come. Hungering and thirsting after righteousness, therefore, must entail a heavenly-mindedness, the Christian hope that looks eagerly for the coming of Christ and full possession of all the benefits of Christ's work. Such a person will be *thinking* about heaven, *longing* for the return of Christ, and *desiring* the attainment of heavenly things. This does not mean that Christians should seek out death or be indifferent to life's responsibilities and joys here and now. But it does mean that they will not readily be trapped by earthly obsessions or caught by death unexpectedly.

Crucial to the cultivation of hope in preparation for death is the practice of prayer. Praying well, that is, praying in the way that Scripture directs us, trains us in hope. The opening petitions of the Lord's Prayer—"hallowed be your name, your kingdom come, your will be done on earth as it is in heaven"—are ultimately requests that Christ would come again, for only then will these things fully come to pass. The Christian who prays the Lord's Prayer with sincerity therefore exercises the virtue of hope. "Come, Lord Jesus" (Rev. 22:20; see 1 Cor. 16:22) is the Christian's biblical, hopeful prayer. Learning to pray well not only prepares us for death because it trains us in the way of hope, but it also prepares us for death because prayer is so important to the dying. The capabilities of dying people are often severely limited. There may be few pleasures and activities left to enjoy. But prayer requires no mobility, appetite, or ability to hear or see. For the dying, prayer may be one of the few things left to do. As with so many other things, prayer is not something that we can neglect during life and then expect to learn in the throes of death. The person who learns to pray through the whole of life is one who is much better prepared for the end of life.

Christians who, by the grace of the Holy Spirit, are cultivating this virtue of hope, and with it a heavenly-minded hunger and thirst for righteousness, will grow into the attitude that Paul describes in 1 Corinthians 7:29–31: "The appointed time has grown very short. From now on, let those who have wives live as though they had none, and those who mourn as though they were not mourning, and those who rejoice as though they were not rejoicing, and those who buy as though they had no goods, and those who deal with the world as though they had no dealings with it. For the present form of this world is passing away." Paul does not counsel us to separate from the world or to despise the world. His words presume that Christians will be marrying, buying, selling, and doing all sorts of other common things. But Christians do so always cognizant of the brevity of life and prepared for life's end.

Love

A way of life that prepares for death must be characterized not only by faith and hope but also by love. Though love ought to characterize the Christian life pervasively, certain aspects of love directly concern preparation for death. It is important to remember that while God alone is the object of our faith and hope, both God and neighbor are the objects of our love. In order to live lives that properly prepare for death, we must grow in the grace of loving our neighbor.

Loving our neighbor presupposes an important fact about human nature: we are social creatures who live in community. A person cannot fulfill the command to love his neighbor if he is seeking to live an isolated life apart from social responsibilities and privileges. God made us, as his image bearers, to live in relationship with him and with our fellow human beings. Thus, to love God and neighbor is to live as God designed us to live. The responsibility to exercise dominion over creation, both in its original form at creation and in its modified form after the fall into sin, requires joint activity and communal endeavors in the many institutions of cultural life. More importantly for Christians, God redeems us by calling us into his church, a community where we hear the Word preached, partake of the sacraments, and enjoy the fellowship of love with fellow believers. Participation in the life of the church is not optional for Christians.

All of this is crucial to keep in mind in the face of various cultural pressures to value independence and even autonomy. People encourage us to plan our lives so that we can attain as much independence as possible—financial or otherwise. To be dependent upon other people is often portrayed as demeaning or pitiful. Is this a proper perspective for Christians? Scripture does indeed warn us about becoming unduly dependent upon others because of laziness or refusal to work. We should strive to be responsible and productive and thereby to provide for our own needs (2 Thess. 3:6–12). One of our motives for such conduct, however, should be the desire to contribute to the needs of others. As social creatures called to love our neighbors we should seek to provide for others in their time of want. Yet being social creatures who love our neighbors also means recognizing that, no matter how hard-working or responsible, *we are and will remain dependent upon others*. We must learn how to *receive* from others as well as how to give. Our pride should not prevent us from accepting help in our own times of need. Our dependence upon others is not demeaning or an insult to our dignity. God made us social creatures and hence mutually dependent creatures, and our true human dignity is expressed in both giving and receiving well, without feelings of arrogant superiority when we are able to give or feelings of (equally arrogant) inferiority when we are in a position to receive.

This task of love—learning to live in communities of mutual dependence with fellow human beings—must be cultivated throughout life. As we do so we are simultaneously preparing for the end of life. The loss of independence is one of the great burdens that many people feel when they are seriously ill and dying. When formerly routine tasks of eating, dressing, and caring for personal hygiene become impossible to accomplish independently in the last stages of life, people become completely reliant upon family, friends, and medical personnel. Understandably, we tend to pity people in such circumstances as those forced to endure great insults to their personal dignity. No one wishes to be unable to do the most basic tasks of life, yet we must keep in mind that being dependent—even *very* dependent—upon others is not in itself an insult to human dignity. Being dependent upon others *well* is in fact one way for us to express our nature as divine image bearers. The handicapped, the disabled, the incapacitated, the seriously ill, and the dying should not be viewed as less than human because of their extraordinary dependence upon others, but as called to be human in ways different from most others.

Of course, none of this means that being in a state of extreme dependence is easy. The fact that it *is* so difficult is the reason why we must strive to learn how to be properly dependent. By learning to live in community with love for our neighbor we prepare ourselves for dying. The person who has cultivated the virtue of love for a long time and thus has learned both to give *and* to receive is much better prepared to face difficult periods of extraordinary dependence upon others. The one who understands that receiving well is a basic human task is better equipped to receive intimate care without seeing it as humiliating or as a violation of human dignity. And that person, released from obsession with her own perceived humiliation, may also be better able to *give* to others in small but significant ways even in times of profound dependence.

Thus far we have focused on the virtue of love as it enables us to receive from and to be dependent upon others, and thereby makes us better prepared for the challenges of dying. But love in its more commonly understood sense—as giving rather than receiving—is also of great value for preparing to die. For one thing, love is important for helping *other* people to die well. Our love for others should prompt genuine concern for the dying and empathy and compassion for those experiencing the spiritual and physical burdens of the end of life.

Some of the practitioners of the *ars moriendi* tradition emphasized the importance of visiting the dying. There are of course many ways in which we can show our love for the dying (such as through writing, calling, praying, preparing meals, or providing financial support), but nothing is quite the same as being with a person. Unfortunately, in the modern world all sorts of hindrances impede the regular practice of visiting the dying. Many recent authors lament the fact that dying has been removed from everyday life. In days past most people died at home, ensconced in a familiar setting and surrounded by family and neighbors who provided whatever care was needed. But in recent years death has been largely institutionalized. Most people who do not die suddenly end up dying in hospitals or in other institutional settings. Medical professionals are often the chief caregivers. The dying, in other words, are taken out of everyday life and sequestered from the people and places that they love. This book is not about public policy, and thus I will not comment on what, if anything, we should do as a society about these realities of modern life. What does concern us here, however, is how to fulfill our responsibilities in love for the dying even in the midst of these new challenges.

To put it simply, the virtue of love compels us to care for the dying in every way possible. Like everyone else, the dying continue to need community, yet in today's world they tend to be particularly isolated. Even if the dying are not living at home, their families should strive to keep them regularly involved in their lives. Churches should continue to treat their dying members as vital parts of the body of Christ, with pastors and elders especially seeking to care for their spiritual needs and deacons for their physical needs. Parents often shelter children from interaction with the dying out of fear that the experience will upset them. But children too should be incorporated, with wisdom, into the regular care offered to the dying. Children also must learn about death and should begin cultivating the virtues that prepare for it. The visiting and caring that family, friends, and churches provide for the dying does not need to have a specific agenda. Generally, Christians ought to "bear one another's burdens" (Gal. 6:2), "encourage the fainthearted, help the weak" (1 Thess. 5:14). We should seek to appreciate (even if we cannot fully understand) the struggles and trials that the dying undergo, and thus seek to build them up in their hope, courage, contentment, patience, and other necessary virtues. Often we may not know what to say. But even then we may remember that on the last day Jesus will say to the blessed: "I was sick and you visited me" (Matt. 25:36).

We care for the dying primarily for their good, not for our own, but we ourselves may experience many benefits when we engage in this practice. For example, when we help to maintain a sense of community for the dying, despite the forces that tend to isolate them, the dying themselves will often be an encouragement to us. They may still give love and not simply receive it. Practicing love toward the dying should also serve to keep the inevitability of our own death before our minds. Contact with those facing imminent death may teach us something of what dying involves and remind us of our own need to prepare for it.

Preparing for Death in Earthly Affairs

Faith, hope, and love play important roles in the Christian's preparation for death. Of course, other virtues, such as courage and contentment, also prepare us to die. To be a person who dies well we must strive to grow in the virtues of the Christian life long before death becomes imminent. But we must also put our earthly affairs in order if we are to die responsibly. This has always been true to some extent. In ages past people recognized the need to "put one's house in order" before death. But the need to attend to earthly affairs has probably been heightened by the increasing complexity of modern life and especially by recent advances in medical technology. The ability to treat many otherwise terminal illnesses and to preserve the lives of those unable to eat, drink, or breathe independently gives us much to be grateful for, but it also raises hitherto unimagined problems. What kind of medical care would I want to receive if I became unable to make decisions for myself? Likewise, many people in developed nations may be thankful for abundant financial resources, yet the complexity of modern financial systems and tax codes also raises hitherto unimagined problems. What will happen to my resources at death, and will my loved ones be provided for in the ways that I intend?

We will later examine difficult decisions about accepting and forgoing medical treatment—both for ourselves and for incapacitated people under our care. First, however, it is important to consider how we ought to prepare for the (not at all remote) possibility that we ourselves might suddenly become incapacitated. How do we wish to be treated, and whom do we wish to make health-care decisions for us? Once we become incapacitated, it is too late to make our wishes known. After considering some of these matters I address some related concerns about financial responsibility, in anticipation of both incapacity and death.

Health Care for the Incapacitated

First, what should we do to prepare for a time when we are in need of medical care but are not able to make decisions for ourselves? How do we ensure, to the best of our ability, that we will be treated in a way that we would wish and that the right people will make necessary decisions for us? The answer is that people may prepare legal documents (often with no attorney required) that give instructions about how they wish to be treated and who will make health-care decisions on their behalf. The precise nature of these documents varies from jurisdiction to jurisdiction, and each reader should check the laws of his own place of residence. In America the individual states regulate these matters, though documents prepared according to the laws of one state are usually recognized in other states, and their instructions are usually followed.

Two principal sorts of documents are the *living will* (or *advance health care directive*) and the *power of attorney for health care*, though states may use somewhat different terms or combine these two into a single document. The basic purpose of the former is to provide instructions about what sort of care a person desires (or does not desire) if she becomes unable to make such decisions. Documents called "living wills" may pertain only to decisions about whether a person wishes to receive life-sustaining treatment when in a permanently unconscious or terminal condition. The ability to give more detailed instructions about a range of possible situations is now commonly available, however, through documents known as "advance health care directives" or something similar. The power of attorney for health care enables a person to name an agent who will have legal authority to make necessary health-care decisions for him when he is in an incapacitated state.

There are numerous reasons why executing such documents is a wise and loving act for nearly every adult. First of all it is for our own good, to ensure that we are treated in ways that we wish when we will have no power to do anything about it. Another reason that may not be as immediately obvious is that preparing such documents is good for our family and others who care about us. When a person becomes incapacitated and in imminent need of health care, loved ones suffer and worry. If we do not leave instructions about how we wish to be cared for, then we may well add to their suffering by keeping them uninvolved or detached from our crisis in ways that they should not be. Another important reason to execute such documents is that they force us to think about the end of life and to discuss its challenges with trusted family members and friends. We ought to be proactive in thinking about the end of life, even though doing this is difficult and unnatural for most people. In order to execute such documents thoughtfully, we are compelled to reflect upon unpleasant scenarios, yet such scenarios are all too possible. If we speak to the person or persons that we name as our agent(s), gaining consent to appoint them and informing them of our wishes, then we create an occasion for having conversations that we would normally avoid. The Bible does not demand that we execute these legal documents. But by initiating such conversations and talking through our options and choices, we follow the way of wisdom, which counsels us to get advice from others before making important decisions.

Once we have made the decision to execute these documents, we face decisions about their content. Appointing an agent is of course a personal decision. We should appoint someone whom we trust and who genuinely cares for us. For many reasons this will ordinarily be a family member. But there may be times, especially when close family members do not share our Christian faith, when choosing a nonfamily member may be the wise course. In any case, the importance of this decision indicates that we should not make it out of a sense of blind duty or sentimentality.

Specifying conditions in which treatments should or should not be administered can be terribly difficult, and I address such issues in the next two chapters rather than here. One general consideration may be useful to mention now, however: wisdom suggests that we should not attempt to micromanage our health-care future but instead should give latitude to the agent whom we appoint. We may be tempted to try to anticipate every possible scenario and to specify what we believe to be the right mode of treatment under each one. Perhaps we do so in order to spare our health-care agent from having to make difficult decisions about us. This sort of thinking, however well intentioned, needs to be challenged. Anticipating future health crises is not easy. There are so many possible circumstances and considerations that it is impossible for anyone to predict what the contours of his own particular situation will be. Consider an analogy from civil law. Legislators ordinarily make laws that state general rules, and judges are expected to apply these laws to specific cases. But some cases involve circumstances that make application of the general rule (seemingly just in itself) unjust in a particular situation. The fact that such cases exist does not mean that there should be no general rules, but it does warn against overconfidence in anticipating all future scenarios.

In the health-care context, heeding this warning suggests the wisdom of giving discretion to our agent. Our agent should be someone who knows us well, who cares for our well-being, and whose wisdom we trust. This agent will be able to see the particular circumstances in which we need care and make judgments accordingly. Is this a burden to our agent, presumably a dear family member or friend? In a sense, yes, but burdening one another is part of what family and friends do. We have responsibilities toward each other, and while we should not *unduly* burden others, taking up a loved one's burdens should be viewed as an act of love, not as an inconsiderate disruption of more important activities. A valued loved one would undoubtedly rather make hard decisions on our behalf than sit by while our own ill-considered instructions are implemented in unforeseen and unfortunate ways.

Finances and the Incapacitated

In addition to these concerns about health care in times of incapacity, we should also strive to put other earthly affairs in order. Finances are an important example. Financial responsibilities vary from person to person, depending upon age, resources, and number of dependents. In general, Scripture counsels parents to provide an inheritance for their children (see 2 Cor. 12:14; Prov. 19:14). Whether or not someone has the resources to provide a large inheritance, everyone must, to the best of his ability, provide for the needs of his dependents. Paul's words are striking: "If anyone does not provide for his relatives, and especially for members of his household, he has denied the faith and is worse than an unbeliever" (1 Tim. 5:8). Even unbelievers ordinarily conduct themselves in this way, so how much worse is it when a believer does not? If we do not wish to burden our loved ones *unduly*, then we need to give attention to such matters. The mere incapacitation or death of a loved one can cause severe hardship for a family, but if the family is also left in financial crisis or has its time consumed by lengthy and unnecessary probate proceedings, then that hardship is only worsened.

Each person must take appropriate steps based upon her own particular situation. Executing a will is imperative for nearly everyone. Many people should take out a life insurance policy as a way of providing immediate financial relief for dependents. Many will also find it helpful to put their financial assets in trusts that will enable their estate to avoid probate, which can often be a long and cumbersome legal process that delays the distribution of an estate's assets. Appointing an agent with power of attorney over financial affairs can also be a wise step to prepare for possible incapacitation. Various laws govern such matters, and they are often complex and murky to the ordinary person. Believers ought to seek help from competent legal and financial professionals in order to arrange their financial affairs effectively.

Showing Love after Death? The Question of Organ Donation

The development of organ transplantation over the past half century has been one of the most astounding accomplishments of modern medicine. Some transplants take place through the gifts of living donors, since it is possible to remove bone marrow, a single kidney, or part of the liver without killing the donor, but first we will consider organ donation at death. We can show love to others even when dying. By dying well a person can set a good example and be an encouragement to those who witness it, and by being financially responsible a person may be able to provide materially for family members or worthy organizations after death. But what about organ donation? Can, or should, a person show love in death not merely by giving spiritual or material gifts to others, but also by agreeing to give a part of one's own body in order to save another's life?

Once again, my purpose is not to resolve public policy disputes, but to examine how a Christian should approach bioethics as part of the broader moral calling of the Christian life. Christians nevertheless have a right to contribute to public policy discussions, and they should thus be aware that many difficult public policy issues exist concerning transplantation. Some of these issues involve matters of supply and demand. How can we procure more organs in order to alleviate long waiting lists for available organs? Should we seek to obtain more organs through free market mechanisms, or perhaps by taking organs from corpses whether or not the person gave consent during life? What is a just way to allocate the organs that are harvested; in other words, how do we decide who receives the organs that become available? How do we prevent the flourishing of black markets in organ donation and reception? Should we pursue xenograft transplants (i.e., harvesting organs for human beings from animals)? In addition to these matters of supply and demand there is the lingering public policy question of when a person should be considered dead. Since it is generally agreed that whole-organ transplants must be taken only from those who have died, how we define the moment of death (in terms of whole-brain, higher-brain, or cardio-pulmonary criteria) is crucial, especially since time is of the essence in harvesting organs from the dead in order to prevent the organs from becoming unusable through the process of ischemia. (I will address the issue of when death occurs in chapter 9.)

Here our concern is with the narrower question of whether individual Christians may or even should agree to become organ donors. It is possible that someday the transplantation system will condone certain sorts of practices that would cause Christians, even if they are not opposed to transplantation in principle, to avoid becoming organ donors or recipients. In the American context today, however, the law prohibits most of the practices that Christians might find most problematic, such as taking whole organs from those who are still alive, taking organs from those who did not give consent (either personally or through their family), experimenting with xenograft transplants, and permitting the buying and selling of organs on the open market. Despite lingering concerns among some Christians about the current understanding of when death has occurred and thus about the morality of certain sorts of organ harvesting, most Christians today can decide whether to become a donor based upon simple questions of principle: is organ transplantation itself morally acceptable? And, if so, do we have a moral obligation to become a donor?

While most Christians today seem to have a positive view of organ donation, there are some genuine objections that could be raised against transplantation from the perspective of Christian theology. For example, is organ transplantation legitimate for creatures created in the image of God? Human beings bear the image of God in both soul and body. We bear the image holistically—that is, no one part of us all by itself can be identified with the image, but we express the image in all aspects of our being. To have hearts, kidneys, and livers is part and parcel of being an image bearer of God, just as having reason and will is. Donating a bodily organ to someone is therefore qualitatively different from doing something for someone or giving money to someone. If I give an irreplaceable part of my body, have I thus violated my status as an image bearer of God? It is worth noting that though the donation is made after death, this question does not really go away. Even after death my body remains *my* body. A corpse is not merely an inanimate thing like a rock, as people recognize across cultures. People would not bother to desecrate graves, nor would other people get repulsed and offended by it, were it not for the fact that human beings tend to identify the dead body with the person whose body it was during life. Corpses are still *named*.

Christian theology gives reason to affirm and reinforce this general human insight. For one thing, Scripture refers to dead bodies as if they still belong to a person. After the crucifixion, for example, Joseph of Arimathea asked for "the body of *Jesus*" (Luke 23:52). The principal theological reason behind this is the fact that the very same body that dies is going to be resurrected one day. The resurrection will not be a creation *ex nihilo* but a transformation of our present mortal bodies: the Lord Jesus Christ "will transform our lowly body to be like his glorious body" (Phil. 3:21). Christian faith, therefore, urges respect for a dead body and prohibits treating it as a warehouse of spare parts for use by others. The dead body does not somehow become the common property of the human race for whatever use it may wish to make of it.

In my judgment these are serious considerations that should probably shape the way in which Christians evaluate future proposals about transplant procedures and policies. But they should not drive us to the conclusion that organ donation and transplantation are sinful per se, for a weighty consideration suggests just the opposite. Christian theology has always taught the goodness of self-sacrifice, even self-sacrifice unto death. God himself showed us the extent of his love by sending his Son to die on our behalf (Rom. 5:8), and as he has done this for us, so the apostle John exhorts us to do this for others: "By this we know love, that he laid down his life for us, and we ought to lay down our lives for the brothers" (1 John 3:16). Since our love for others ought to extend even to the point of death, the argument that we should never do anything that would endanger our bodily integrity is faulty. Christlike love for our neighbor involves willingness to suffer the dissolution of body and soul, the greatest imaginable assault upon our image-bearing nature. Giving up an organ postmortem for another person is a less radical act than giving up one's life for another. Donating an organ after death does not destroy life, disrupt the soul's communion with God in heaven, or interfere with God's ability to raise our bodies unto a whole, perfect, and glorified state on the last day. If God is able to raise the bodies of his martyrs who have been torn and eaten by lions, then he is certainly able to raise the bodies of Christians who have donated a heart or liver to a suffering human being. Provided that the dead bodies are treated respectfully, and that organs are genuinely *given* rather than *taken*, Christians, having received in Christ the greatest token of self-giving love imaginable, have good reason to view organ donation as a charitable act of self-giving.

Christians, therefore, *may* consent to donate organs after death. But *must* Christians do so? Especially in light of the long waiting lists for organs and the dismal prognosis for those who do not receive transplants in a timely way, do Christians have an obligation to donate? Such a conclusion may seem warranted from the verse in 1 John 3 that immediately follows the exhortation to lay down our lives for our brothers: "If anyone has the world's goods and sees his brother in need, yet closes his heart against him, how does God's love abide in him?" (1 John 3:17).

Nevertheless, other considerations suggest caution before laying upon believers an absolute obligation to donate. Paul's discussion of giving in 2 Corinthians 8–9 is instructive. He calls upon the Corinthian Christians to overflow with generosity toward their fellow believers. But he never places any precise obligation upon them, in noticeable contrast to the Old Testament, which has specific rules for required gifts, such as the tithe. Paul's chief wish was for giving "bountifully," and he called for each one to "give as he has decided in his heart, not reluctantly or under compulsion, for God loves a cheerful giver" (2 Cor. 9: 7). If this is the case with lesser gifts, such as money, how much more must this be true with greater gifts such as an organ from one's body? If we may not lay absolute obligations for giving external, material gifts upon other Christians, then surely we must refrain from laying absolute obligations for giving body parts. Christians should be exhorting each other to be generous, but we should leave the precise shape of each person's generosity to her own discretion. Each believer has the Christian liberty to be generous according to the measure of grace given by God. Not that this gives us an easy excuse to refuse to become organ donors. Decisions to give or not to give money, or to donate or not to donate organs, should be undertaken thoughtfully, and good reasons should underlie the choices that we make. In light of the great need for donated organs and the simplicity of consenting to be a donor, I believe that Christians should be generally eager to give such consent, though they need not answer to one another about their decisions in this area.

The same sort of reasoning seems appropriate when considering the donation of a renewable part of our body, such as bone marrow. Given the ease of becoming registered in the National Bone Marrow Registry and the very real possibility that one could prove to be an appropriate match for someone whose life depends upon a bone marrow transplant, compelling considerations suggest that Christians should be eager to participate. Yet again this is a decision that each person makes before God, not in order to answer to a fellow believer. Other cases, such as becoming a living organ donor (of a kidney or partial liver), place a significant burden upon the donor because of the risk of serious injury or even death. These are morally harrowing cases and require us to be even more studious in avoiding quick judgments about other people's decisions.

Conclusion

Psalm 90 instructs us to number our days that we may gain a heart of wisdom. With that goal in mind we have examined how Christians should view their own future death and how they ought to prepare for it throughout life, through pursuing virtue, putting their earthly affairs in order, and considering how their bodies might be given as gifts to others when they die. We do not know when we will die, whether sooner or later, gradually or suddenly. But we do know that we will die one day if the Lord does not return first, and in anticipation of that unknown day we are called to take responsibility for our lives now, becoming the sort of people who will die well and will bless others in our death. Though dying will not be easy, preparing well offers promise of much gain for ourselves and other people—and will bring glory to God. In the final two chapters we will consider some of the difficult choices that people must make about death, not when it is still far away and there is opportunity to prepare, but when death seems near. We must consider how we should evaluate the common distinction between killing and letting die, and how our conclusion affects the decisions we make—for ourselves and others—about accepting and refusing medical treatment at the end of life.

8

SUICIDE, EUTHANASIA, AND THE DISTINCTION BETWEEN KILLING AND LETTING DIE

In chapter 7 we considered the Christian's calling to live with death in view. The whole of the Christian life ought to be structured in light of the fact that we all must die someday. Yet we do not know when that day will be. In order to die well, therefore, Christians of all ages must set their faith and hope in Christ and seek to cultivate all of the virtues, so that death will not find them unprepared to face the trials and sufferings of the end of life or unprepared to meet their Creator.

The *ars moriendi* literature flourished at a time when life expectancy was much shorter than today and when most people died at home, surrounded by family, after relatively short illnesses. Today most people live much longer lives, but many of them spend those extra years not in their homes but in institutional settings, and many of them die not after short illnesses but after a protracted aging process during which medical technology preserves an increasingly feeble and uncomfortable earthly life. Medical advancements have produced the cure for many diseases and have extended life expectancy, yet they have not banished death. Ironically, they have managed to *increase* many people's anxieties about the end of life. The well-publicized legal struggles over the proper treatment of Karen Ann Quinlan, Nancy Cruzan, and Terry Schiavo have showcased the troubling moral issues that our medical technology has spawned. The moving book and film, *The Diving Bell and the Butterfly*, have given us startling insight into the experience of "locked-in syndrome" and the possibility of being kept alive with a perfectly functioning mind and an almost totally inert body. Those sorts of cases are still rare, but people now know that being preserved from death in order to live miserable, pitiful, or even unconscious lives is a very real possibility. We continue to marvel at each new medical advance, yet often shudder to contemplate being a recipient of such advances—at least for too long and under the wrong circumstances. The longer life can be preserved, it seems, the more interest people show in death "with dignity."

Who does not desire a dignified death? Yet for many people "death with dignity" has come to mean a "right to die"—and even a right to receive help from a physician in committing suicide. The question of the morality of suicide is certainly not new. Thousands of years ago many famous figures of classical Greece and Rome praised suicide as a way of avoiding dishonor or a painful death. With the expansion of Christianity in the Western world, suicide came under almost universal condemnation, but various voices have called for a rethinking of this position in recent centuries. The modern interest in human rights and related ideas about personal autonomy and the mastery of nature provided impetus for the advocacy of euthanasia. Combined with increasing prospects for living long but uncomfortable lives due to new medical technology, claims about a right to die have taken on special strength in recent decades. People such as Jack Kevorkian, the Michigan physician, and Derek Humphry, founder of the Hemlock Society, have become widely known advocates of the right to die; and the legalization of physician-assisted suicide (PAS) under prescribed conditions in Oregon and especially in the Netherlands has attracted considerable attention. While most Christian writers have spoken critically of PAS and the so-called right to die, they have also tended to resist contemporary expectations that illness should be combated and life extended whenever technologically possible.

These developments raise pressing and difficult bioethical questions. A host of public policy issues revolve around what obligations we have to extend life and what rights we have to end it, and Christians may participate in debates about these issues. I examine these questions not as public policy problems, however, but from the perspective of the believer seeking to live a faithful Christian life. Whatever the social trends of the future may be, Christians have the responsibility to think through, in light of the work of Christ and their faith in him, how they ought to view the alleged right to die and how they ought to make decisions about when to accept and when to refuse medical treatment. We must consider the issue of suicide, PAS, and the controversial distinction between *killing* and *letting die*. After defending the legitimacy and importance of this distinction between killing and letting die, we will consider how Christians should resolve difficult decisions about treatment (and nontreatment) options. To affirm that it may be morally permissible to let oneself or another person die still leaves the difficult question of *when* such a choice is rightly made. In all of these discussions we must keep before us the basic Christian affirmations that life is a divine gift, that death is a great enemy, and that our heavenly inheritance is the most profound hope of all.

Suicide and the Christian Life

The controversies about euthanasia and PAS—and even some questions about accepting and refusing treatment—take us back to basic questions about suicide. Does a person have a right to take his own life, at least in certain circumstances? Most people, including Christians, recoil at the thought of one person killing another person, but at the same time they affirm broad rights for individuals to choose the sort of lives they wish to live and to do as they wish with their own property. Many have suggested that rights to choose a way of life and to dispose of property logically ought to extend to decisions about ending life. Does a person not have a property right in his own body? If a person has the right to choose a way of life, does he not have the right to end his life?

Christians have traditionally rejected this logic. I believe that they have been correct to do so, but it is worth asking why. Simplistic answers are tempting and perhaps instinctively attractive, but weak explanations for why we should reject suicide as a moral right are counterproductive and ought to be rejected. In opposing the right to commit suicide, for example, Christians sometimes respond by affirming that we should not "play God" or stand opposed to God's will. Yet we make decisions and take responsibility for matters all the

time without thinking that we are thereby usurping divine authority. Ultimately everything that comes to pass happens according to
God's will, yet that does not relieve us of responsibility for our moral
choices. We would never condemn the person who rescues someone
drowning in a pool, as if that person has usurped God's authority
over life and death.

Biblical Teaching about Suicide

An examination of Scripture, nevertheless, indicates that there is
something fundamentally correct about the Christian's instinct to
condemn suicide as an attempt to control what has not been placed
in human hands. Ecclesiastes teaches that there is "a time to be born,
and a time to die . . ." (Eccles. 3:2) but also reminds us that "no man has
power to retain the spirit, or power over the day of death . . ." (Eccles.
8:8). "When the time drew near that Israel must die" (Gen. 47:29),
he did not fight that inevitable event but recognized its approach and
acted accordingly. While this does not mean that there is never a time
to fight off the threat of death, Scripture reminds us that, as with the
beginning of life, there is something mysterious and profound about
the end of life. The end of life ultimately transcends human control and shows us the limits of human capabilities. Whatever rightful
responsibility we should take in regard to matters of life and death,
we must do so carefully, mindful not to tamper with the boundaries
that God has established.

These boundaries are most evidently traced by God in his simple
command, enshrined in the Decalogue and repeated many other places
in Scripture: "You shall not kill." Human beings may not take human
life. The general way in which this commandment is stated suggests
that there is no morally crucial distinction between taking another
person's life and taking one's own. Suicide is a form of homicide. This
initial conclusion is correct, in my judgment, but it is complicated by
two facts: Scripture presents exceptions to the general prohibition
of killing, and Scripture never explicitly condemns suicide. Each of
these complications is worth examining briefly.

First, what are the exceptions to the general command not to kill,
and might suicide be properly categorized as an exception to the
rule? Scripture itself points to three sorts of situations in which killing
another person is permitted and sometimes even obligatory. These
three exceptional situations are also broadly (though not universally)

recognized by people of other faiths and encoded in many civil legal systems. Killing is justified when administering capital punishment, when waging (a just) war, and when defending one's own or another's life (e.g., see Gen. 9:6; 14:1–16; Ex. 22:2–3). Why these three particular cases? That is, what is it about these three situations that justifies taking life in the face of the strong divine prohibition against killing? The answer to this question helps us to answer the question whether suicide is another legitimate exception.

The common denominator that connects the three exceptional situations—capital punishment, war, and defense of life—is that they all spring directly out of *profound respect* for the sixth commandment itself. All of them reflect the positive side of the sixth commandment: the sanctity of human life and the duty to preserve and protect it. Killing is permitted in these situations, in other words, because of our horror about the act of killing. The one crime that Scripture declares universally worthy of capital punishment is *murder* (Gen. 9:6). Warfare is justly conducted only when it is pursued not in order to conquer but in order to defend against a hostile enemy who threatens innocent life (I understand God's command to Israel to wage "holy war" against the residents of Canaan to be unique and therefore not a model for anyone today). Killing in self-defense is legitimate only when it aims to protect a person's *life*, not his property or reputation. What this means is that apparent violations of the sixth commandment are permissible or even obligatory when the purposes of *the sixth commandment itself* are at stake. When exercised properly, capital punishment, warfare, and killing in defense of life uphold the moral goals of the sixth commandment rather than impede them—though such situations are indeed tragic.

How does suicide compare to these three exceptional situations? Can suicide be added to our list of exceptions? The answer is no. While capital punishment, warfare, and killing in self-defense, when performed justly, serve to defend and vindicate life, suicide only destroys it. Of course, we can imagine situations in which people kill themselves in order to save another's life. For example, someone might throw herself on the tracks in front of an oncoming train, not for the purpose of ending her own life but in order to push aside an unconscious person lying on the track. But such scenarios are not ordinarily considered acts of suicide. Suicide occurs when a person decides to end his life because of its perceived misery or hopelessness, and this advances no good purpose of the sixth commandment. For this reason, suicide is fundamentally different from the situations that constitute legitimate exceptions to the general command not to kill. Christians ought to live in such a way that upholds the purposes of the sixth commandment—by not killing if possible and by taking life in exceptional circumstances—but the act of suicide runs in precisely the opposite direction.

The second complication of applying "do not kill" to the case of suicide, as mentioned above, is the fact that Scripture never explicitly condemns suicide. If suicide is indeed a serious sin—self-murder—then why this silence? One possible answer is that suicide is so obviously contrary to broader biblical teaching about human nature and human moral responsibility that an explicit prohibition is unnecessary. This response is plausible, but lest we be left with any lingering suspicion that the Bible takes an ambiguous stance toward suicide, a brief look at the several cases of suicide recounted in Scripture should leave little doubt that it is presented in a decidedly negative light.

All five people whom Scripture records as committing suicide were wicked men, and in at least several cases Scripture portrays their suicides as tragically fitting ends to self-destructive, downward-spiraling lives. The first biblically recorded suicide is that of Abimelech (Judg. 9:54). Judges 9 portrays Abimelech in a negative light from the outset, reporting that he killed his seventy brothers on one stone in a shocking but successful bid to secure power over a part of Israel (Judg. 9:5–6). The events leading to Abimelech's death (actually an assisted suicide, since his armor-bearer killed him upon his orders) are introduced as God's designed way to punish him for murdering his brothers (Judg. 9:23–24). After his assisted suicide, which he pursued to avoid the shame of being killed by a woman, Scripture remarks: "Thus God returned the evil of Abimelech . . ." (Judg. 9:56). Death by suicide, therefore, reflected the judgment of God. The second example is similar. First Samuel presents the story of Israel's first king, Saul, as one of initial promise that quickly and precipitously falls into disaster. Saul turns out to be rebellious, foolish, self-serving, and violent. He repeatedly attempts to kill David, who had served him faithfully, and the penultimate event of Saul's life is the deplorable act of seeking divine counsel through a witch (1 Samuel 28). As Saul sinks to ever new lows, 1 Samuel ends with the climax of the king's decline: his suicide (1 Sam. 31:4).

Two of the other biblically recorded suicides look very similar to each other, and intentionally so. Both Ahithophel and Judas Iscariot were close associates of their masters, David and Jesus the Son of David, respectively. Both became traitors, Ahithophel aiding Absolam in his coup against David and Judas guiding the chief priests in their capture of Jesus. And both, in despair at the turn of events, hanged themselves (2 Sam. 17:23; Matt. 27:5). In the case of these two, therefore, as with Abimelech and Saul, Scripture presents suicide in an unambiguously negative light, as the fitting end of a wicked and unrepentant life. The remaining biblical example confirms this conclusion. First Kings 16 relates how Zimri became king of Israel as a traitor, rising up in treason against King Elah. Zimri has the distinction of having the shortest reign of any Israelite king—a mere seven days—and his reign ended when he burned a house around him in order to avoid capture (1 Kings 16:18). Why did Zimri's life come to such an end? "Because of his sins that he committed, doing evil in the sight of the LORD . . ." (1 Kings 16:19). Suicide, once again, is a human act that serves as a means of divine retribution following great sins.

This consistently negative portrayal of suicide in Scripture is thrown into sharper relief by a biblical story in which a godly man is lured toward a suicidal act but refuses on moral and theological grounds. God's description of this man, Job, stands in stark contrast to the biblical verdicts about Abimelech, Saul, Ahithophel, Zimri, and Judas: "There is none like him on the earth, a blameless and upright man, who fears God and turns away from evil" (Job 1:8). It is not as if Job's sufferings were slight. Job 1–2 records how Satan, with God's permission, took away the bulk of Job's wealth, secured the death of all of his children, and afflicted him with painful sores from head to foot. Job would be a prime candidate for suicide, and his wife suggested just such a course: "Do you still hold fast your integrity? Curse God and die" (Job 2:9). It is unclear how exactly Job's wife envisioned that his death would occur after rejecting God, but she urges him to pursue a course suicidal in nature, in which death would follow as a result of his own action. Job, however, despite the deep despair that he would express repeatedly in the following chapters, rejected his wife's proposal out of hand: "You speak as one of the foolish women would speak. Shall we receive good from God, and shall we not receive evil?" Hence the biblical verdict follows: "In all this Job did not sin with his lips" (Job 2:10). Perhaps most remarkable here is that Job

associates himself shortly thereafter with those "who long for death
. . . who . . . are glad when they find the grave" (Job 3:21–22). In his
suffering he desired to die at times, yet as a godly man Job refused to
bring about death by his own hand.

Suicide in the Light of Image Bearing and Righteous Suffering

These considerations indicate that Christians have been correct to
condemn suicide as a violation of the sixth commandment. A few
other moral and theological considerations strengthen this conclusion by putting it into broader perspective. These considerations
relate to the Christian's calling to live a socially responsive life as an
image bearer of God and to endure suffering righteously under God's
benevolent providence.

First, God's creation of human beings in his own image means that
we are inherently social creatures and entails a responsibility to live not
as independent, isolated individuals but as members of communities
with mutual obligations. What one person does affects many others.
Except in the rare case of someone who genuinely lacks family and
friends, a person who commits suicide leaves people behind who are
deeply grieved by his death and often plagued by guilt about what
they might have done to prevent it. A family not only loses one of its
members, but surviving family members sometimes also see their own
relationships strained as a result of this act. Advocates of the right to
die often base their case on individual rights and the autonomy of the
patient. But the claim that our lives are our own and that the decision
to preserve life or to end life is an expression of autonomous choice is
hardly consistent either with a biblical theology of the image of God
or with our experience of real life and the devastating consequences
of suicide upon many people.

Second, the prohibition of suicide should be seen in the light of the
Christian's calling to suffer righteously under the benevolent providence of God. This consideration reflects the fact that most suicides
occur in response to or in expectation of great suffering. Though
suicide is not a problem limited to any particular group—young or
old, male or female, or particular ethnic group—the one thing that
most people who take their own lives share in common is a history
of depression. On the one hand, this fact ought to qualify the way
that we condemn suicide as a serious sin. In rejecting the right to

take one's own life, our attitude toward those expressing suicidal tendencies should not be judgmental but compassionate. Christian love commends a merciful approach to those who are struggling with great anguish and despair, whatever the cause (and most likely it is complex). Suicide is a sin and must be dealt with as such, but it is not the unforgivable sin that automatically condemns a person to hell, as some Christian theologians have taught.

On the other hand, the fact that so many incidences of suicide are linked to a history of depression prompts us to reflect upon our view of suffering. How should those who are suffering greatly respond in a way consistent with Christian faith? As considered in chapter 2, suffering is not something that is optional or avoidable in the present life. Our Lord endured the cross and has called his followers to take up the cross in fellowship with him (Matt. 16:24–25). Paul reminds us that we are children of God and fellow heirs with Christ, "provided we suffer with him in order that we may also be glorified with him" (Rom. 8:17). The present life is not one of earthly glory and conquest. Instead, Christians must look to the age to come as the fulfillment of those desires, for as Paul goes on to say: "The sufferings of this present time are not worth comparing with the glory that is to be revealed to us" (Rom. 8:18). Suffering is a constituent part of the Christian life, and Christians are called to be people of hope and joy and gratitude *in the midst of* their suffering, not merely when suffering is absent. Again, the story of Job is greatly encouraging. Job suffered profoundly and at times spoke precipitously, but he refused to give up by embracing death (Job 2:9–10), he remained steadfast (James 5:11), and he was ultimately commended by God (Job 42:7). God never did tell Job exactly why he had to suffer when and how he did, but he did set before him his greatness and wisdom—just because Job did not know the reasons for his suffering does not mean that God did not know! And in the fullness of time we have seen God's ultimate answer to the question of suffering, not in the form of a philosophical answer but in the death and resurrection of his Son, in whom suffering and death have been experienced and overcome.

In response to suffering that made him at times long for death, then, Job the righteous man *humbled* himself before God (Job 42:2–6) and remained *steadfast* (James 5:11). What a different sort of attitude this is in comparison to the claims made by many advocates of a right to die. The proper Christian response to great suffering is not the assertion of autonomy or dignity, but humility and steadfastness in the face of despair. There are earthly remedies that may be sought by those and for those who are suffering, such as medical care for illnesses and, with caution, antidepressant medication that can stave off desperate measures for many people and return them to a functional state. Those contemplating the end of life with anxiety can be comforted by the fact that modern analgesics make nearly all experiences of pain manageable, such that no one need die today in great physical anguish. But Christians must look at these earthly blessings as temporal and transient. The physical care that can alleviate some suffering must be accompanied by spiritual care that points the beleaguered of this world to the Lord Jesus Christ who suffered like them and for them, and who as their great high priest is able and willing to help them (Heb. 2:17–18)—not by taking away all suffering now but by pouring out blessings upon them in the present age (such as the Holy Spirit and the church, with their ministry of Word and sacrament) and a firm and unshakable hope for the age to come (1 Pet. 1:3–7).

Physician-Assisted Suicide

This discussion of suicide prompts consideration of the controversial issue of physician-assisted suicide. Suicide, however morally problematic, is no longer prohibited by law in the Western world. But assisting someone in committing suicide generally remains illegal, though there are a few noteworthy exceptions to this rule. This suggests that PAS raises some distinct moral issues from those raised by suicide in general.

For the sake of clarity we should examine a few points of terminology and definition. In common parlance, "euthanasia" is often roughly identified with PAS, though the terms are not synonymous. "Euthanasia" literally means "good death," which is not particularly helpful in establishing a useful definition. In the present day, euthanasia ordinarily refers to one person deliberately bringing about the death of another person who (at least in many cases) has been diagnosed with a terminal illness. It is important to note that such an act is not performed out of malicious motives but out of benevolent motives, and hence constitutes a form of "mercy killing." Though euthanasia as so defined encompasses involuntary killing (that is, not requested by the suffering patient), those who advocate the legalization of euthanasia ordinarily insist that it should be performed only upon those who are rational and competent and who specifically request it. Some writers make a distinction between *active* euthanasia and *passive* euthanasia. The former refers to doing something to a person that brings about his death (such as giving a lethal injection) and the latter refers to the deliberate withholding of something from a person that is necessary to sustain life. Later I will discuss the related distinction between killing and letting die, as well as how we should make decisions about when forgoing treatment is proper. For now, however, I suggest limiting "euthanasia" to the so-called active euthanasia, so as not to confuse this course of action with decisions to forgo treatment. Strictly speaking, "assisted suicide" occurs when one person aids another person in taking his own life. Since physicians are well equipped to provide the means for a quick and painless death, such as by lethal injection, *physician*-assisted suicide has become a matter of particular interest.

For many Christians, the question of PAS may seem rather simple. If suicide is morally wrong, then soliciting someone's help to perform suicide and aiding a person in committing suicide seem impossible to justify. The biblical cases of Abimelech and Saul considered earlier support this intuition. Their attempts to solicit assistance in ending their own lives do not seem morally different from the direct suicidal acts of figures such as Ahithophel and Judas.

But in real life things often look much more complicated. Those looking for help in ending their lives seldom seem to be defiantly seeking to usurp the prerogatives of God. Instead, they are people who suffer greatly, who feel weighty burdens and anxieties, and who are sincerely in search of help. It is often our best Christian instincts that cause us to sympathize with and to withhold blame from these people who want to end such a difficult life. Thus how ought Christians to respond to those who desire PAS? Christians, of all people, should be merciful toward the suffering, but in the case of PAS we must think carefully about what constitutes mercy. If the suffering person is not a believer, then supporting a desire to hasten death is in effect encouraging a person to come into the presence of God apart from Christ. Surely this is no expression of true love and compassion and no answer at all for the hardship of suffering. If the suffering person is a believer, then what she needs to hear is the comfort and encouragement of the gospel that she professes. We must remind her that she has a merciful High Priest in heaven whom she may approach now, in the midst of her sufferings, and who is continually interceding for her (see Heb. 2:17–18; 4:14–16; 7:25). God promises that no matter how great the temptation is, he will provide a way out (1 Cor. 10:13). Enabling suicide is encouraging a person to think that there is no answer to her despair, no available comfort in her present affliction—directly the opposite of what the gospel proclaims. True compassion exhibits itself in appropriate assistance. But giving or receiving assistance in suicide hardly befits those who belong to Jesus Christ.

Beyond such concerns about personal Christian conduct in the face of PAS lie a number of controversial public policy matters. For most people, the moral status of PAS determines whether or not it should be legal. Some writers, nevertheless, though morally troubled by PAS, support the right of other people to pursue it while others, though open to the moral legitimacy of PAS in some circumstances, oppose its legalization because of negative social effects. I do not intend to delve deeply into the public policy dimensions of this issue. A few considerations, however, may be worth mentioning for the benefit of Christians who will be engaging in public policy debates about PAS. First, experiments with legalized PAS have brought to light many potential abuses. In the Netherlands, for example, studies have shown that a great many instances of PAS have gone unreported (contrary to legal requirement) and have raised concerns that the practice of *involuntary* euthanasia is not uncommon. Second, the usual insistence that PAS should only be legal in cases when the patient is rational and competent is a safeguard that may be much better in theory than in practice. The strong correlation of suicidal tendencies with a history of depression raises questions about how sure we can be that a person requesting PAS truly makes a decision emerging out of rational reflection rather than out of severe emotional despair. Third, many writers have eloquently expressed concern about what the legalization of PAS threatens to do to the medical profession. Changing the long Western tradition of seeing physicians as healers who refuse to deal out death and presenting physicians instead as those who both preserve life *and* bring death, upon the patient's request, has the potential for far-reaching implications for the conduct and public perception of the medical profession.

Killing and Letting Die

We can conclude that though Christians should be compassionate rather than judgmental toward those struggling with suicidal temptations, suicide is a serious sin that violates the sixth commandment. Perhaps lingering in the back of many readers' minds through this discussion, however, is this question: if taking my own life is morally prohibited, must I take every possible measure at all times to preserve life? In other words, granted that I should not take positive steps to bring about my own death, is it ever permissible or even obligatory to forgo medical treatment that promises to extend life and thus to allow death to take me earlier than it might otherwise? As commonly put, this question asks whether there is a meaningful moral distinction between *killing* (prohibited) and *letting die* (potentially permissible or obligatory).

The idea that there must be at least *some* situations when forgoing treatment is a morally righteous decision strikes a strong chord with most Christians. A few initial considerations indicate why that is the case. Most broadly, Scripture teaches that our present earthly life is not the highest good. Our future, heavenly life is of much greater importance, and God turns death, though an enemy, into a blessing for Christians in significant respects. If this is the case, then the view teaching that earthly life should be preserved at any cost (sometimes referred to as "vitalism") seems contrary to Christian faith and hope. Jesus instills this conviction in his followers: "Whoever finds his life will lose it, and whoever loses his life for my sake will find it" (Matt. 10:39). This perspective lies behind several biblical examples that, though nonmedical in nature, illustrate that Christians should willingly give up earthly life in certain circumstances. Self-sacrifice unto death is not only permissible for the Christian, but even commended: "By this we know love, that he laid down his life for us, and we ought to lay down our lives for the brothers" (1 John 3:16). Martyrdom offers another example. Allegiance to Christ and profession of the gospel are more important than preserving earthly life, and thus many Christians through history have refused to forsake their Lord for the sake of preserving their earthly lives as long as possible. As Paul said, "I am ready not only to be imprisoned but even to die in Jerusalem for the name of the Lord Jesus" (Acts 21:13).

These initial considerations are probably quite weighty for most Christians. But very intelligent and persuasive people have argued that despite widespread acceptance of the basic distinction between killing and letting die, there is no true moral difference between them. Examining their claims is helpful for understanding the importance of this distinction and its usefulness for confronting the kinds of choices to be explored in the next chapter.

One of the most frequently discussed arguments rejecting the moral distinction between killing and letting die is offered by philosopher James Rachels. Rachels argues that a physician is responsible for death in either case—whether he brings death actively or fails to act such that death occurs when he could have prevented it. In both cases the physician does something, either taking initiative to bring death or letting death occur. Neither act is necessarily right or wrong. Either action is wrong if death is a bad thing in a given circumstance, and either is right if death is a good thing in a given circumstance. The mere difference between killing and letting die is therefore morally indifferent, Rachels concludes, and the moral crux of the issue is whether death is a good thing in a particular concrete situation. Rachels illustrates his point by imagining two scenarios. Both scenarios involve people who wish to kill a child for identical reasons. In one scenario the person goes into the room where the child is taking a bath and holds the child's head under the water until he dies. In the other scenario the person, when entering the room, finds that the child has just hit his head, become unconscious, and sunk under water. Instead of lifting the child out of the water he simply leaves the room. Rachels argues that these two men were driven by the same motives, accomplished the same goal, and are equally morally responsible for the child's death. The crucial issue is that this innocent child's death was a bad thing, and the way in which it was accomplished (actively killing or passively letting die) is morally indifferent.

Rachels's argument has an initial appeal, but it has crucial flaws, and there are compelling reasons to maintain the important moral distinction between killing and letting die. I would concede that there are certain circumstances in which a decision to kill actively and a decision to let someone die when it is in our power to prevent it are equally morally reprehensible. The example of the child in the bathtub may well be an example of this. In the medical context, we might imagine a doctor who dislikes a patient and wants her dead, despite the fact that she desires to be healed and has a curable illness. We would probably condemn this doctor just as strongly if he intentionally withheld a treatment necessary to prevent her death as if he secretly gave her a lethal injection. But even in such carefully constructed scenarios in which the moral guilt attaching to two different courses of action seems to be equal, the two different courses of actions *themselves* are not the same. If one of my neighbors shouts an insult at me from across the street and another neighbor steals a flowerpot from my front yard, I might judge that they have wronged me in equally serious ways. But I would not therefore conclude that there is no meaningful moral distinction to be made between insulting and stealing. They are different moral actions and require a different moral analysis for understanding and evaluating them properly.

The same thing is true, I suggest, with the distinction between killing and letting die. Actively bringing about a person's death—by drowning, lethal injection, or whatever—is quite simply not the same thing as deciding not to intervene when something else is bringing death upon a person. One of the most important reasons why this is the case is that death is a force that exists independent of human agency. Despite the pretensions of modern medical technology, human beings did not invent death nor can they eliminate it. Daniel Callahan has written eloquently on this point, arguing that we need to recover a sense of *nature*. Equating killing and letting die is tantamount to making *all* death the fault of human beings, as if dying from cancer and being murdered must both be assigned to human fault. Dying from cancer, in this way of thinking, is the result of a failure in medical technology while being murdered is a failure in law enforcement. From a Christian perspective, Callahan's point should be modified to some degree. Ultimately all death *is* the fault of human beings, since Scripture ascribes to Adam's first sin the blame for the reign of death (Gen. 2:17; 3:19; Rom. 5:12; 6:23). But once we move beyond ascribing human fault to death *in general* and inquire into guilt for *particular* deaths, the distinction between killing and letting die is crucial if we are to make any sense of the world. In the confines of this present age, there are things that we can do to reduce the occurrence of murder, that is, the active taking of people's lives. But there is nothing that we can do to eliminate death. Even if we were to reduce the murder rate to zero, everybody would still die. Improvements in medical technology might succeed in pushing back the average age of death, but the death rate would remain 100 percent. In light of this reality, to deny that there is a meaningful moral distinction between letting someone die of "natural causes" and actively taking someone's life before nature can take its course is highly unsatisfactory. If the basic theological point made earlier is true—namely, that the day of death is ultimately God's prerogative—then to act as if man is the ultimate master of death by equating killing and letting die is fundamentally problematic from a Christian perspective.

Callahan and others conclude that erasing these crucial distinctions and acting as though we are the masters of death tends to create a kind of slavery to our medical technology. In dethroning God and the natural order we end up slaves to the work of our own hands. Our medical technology, which was designed to be of service to us and for our good, threatens to enslave us to its demands. If there is no meaningful distinction between killing and letting die, and if they are both morally wrong, then we are obligated to use whatever technology is available to us to preserve life in every situation, whatever the circumstances, lest we become guilty of murder. If we have the technology to do something, in other words, we must use it. Yet if we seek to avoid this conclusion by asserting that there is no meaningful distinction between killing and letting die, and that they are both permissible, then the door is opened wide for suicide, PAS, and euthanasia of all sorts. To deny this important distinction, therefore, leaves us with regrettable and ironic moral options.

Another consideration that may help us to appreciate the moral distinction between killing and letting die is the fact that with the former we are necessarily aiming at death as our goal while with the latter this is not necessarily (and usually not) the case. To kill—that is, actively to take someone's life—is by definition to choose death, whether this be done out of wicked or merciful motives. To let an ill person die (ourselves or another), however, may well be to choose not death but one form of life over another. A person's choice to forgo an additional round of chemotherapy when her cancer is evidently a terminal case is probably not a choice to die. The fact of death has already been decided, apart from the cancer victim's will. Instead, the choice to forgo more chemotherapy may be a decision to *live* a somewhat shorter life than the chemotherapy might make possible, but a shorter life that is free from the debilitating burden of chemotherapy and that enables the person to enjoy her remaining life more—to finish projects, to spend time with loved ones, and to get her house in order. It is not necessarily a choice between life and death, therefore, but a choice between one kind of life and another kind of life. The fact is, we constantly make choices among various kinds of life, some of which increase the odds that our lives will be shorter than they otherwise might be. By choosing to drive cars we decide to live a kind of life that we deem better than the kind of life that we would lead if we never drove, despite the fact that driving increases the odds of dying a premature death. By choosing to be a firefighter, a person decides to live a certain kind of life that carries greater risks of a premature death than most other occupations, yet no one would claim that such a career decision is a choice of death over life.

Returning to the bioethical context, we can see that the moral choice to let die can be vastly different from the moral choice to kill. The choice to kill is a choice to bring death, a choice against life. But the choice to let die by refusing additional chemotherapy is not a choice to bring death—cancer is bringing death however much one wishes it would not. In the face of death, the choice to forgo treatment may still be a choice about how to live.

A final point addresses a danger about which a number of writers have warned. This danger is that equating killing and letting die puts pressure on people to keep patients alive as long as possible, which in turn tends to increase the demand for PAS and other forms of euthanasia. What begins as a seemingly high view of life ends up catalyzing a lower view of life. The reason for this irony is twofold. First, the longer and more aggressively we seek to preserve the lives of the feeble, incapacitated, and dying, and thus the less we let disease and old age take their natural course, the more people we bring into physically miserable states of life, thus creating fertile soil for appeals for euthanasia to relieve such people from their misery. Second, the equation of killing and letting die corresponds to a mindset that implicitly imputes control over life and death to human beings rather than to God and his natural order. It is precisely such a mindset that promotes the assertion of a right to die according to one's autonomous choice. If man is indeed the master of life and death, then denying the right to PAS will be a hard sell.

Conclusion

The recent explosion of medical technology that has greatly enhanced our ability to prolong life, combined with the modern emphasis upon individual rights, has produced considerable social pressure to recognize a right to die and a right to receive help in dying, for the purpose of escaping end-of-life suffering and attaining an elusive death with dignity. Despite the sympathy that Christians often feel toward such demands when they contemplate the genuine misery that many people experience in their last days, the theological and ethical truths of Christianity highlight the incompatibility of suicide with Christian faith and life. These truths redirect, in directions other than suicide, our proper desire to show compassion and mercy toward those who are suffering. Nevertheless, opposition to suicide and PAS should not blind us to the genuine and important distinction between killing and letting die. While the former is always wrong, the latter may be a morally permissible or even compelling decision.

But these conclusions leave outstanding the very difficult question of how to evaluate the various situations that fall into the category of letting die. When is forgoing treatment right, and when is it wrong? To these questions we turn in the final chapter.

9

ACCEPTING AND FORGOING TREATMENT

In chapter 8 I argued for the importance of the moral distinction between killing and letting die, but I ended by asking a question that I did not answer: when is the choice to let die—that is, to forgo further treatment—morally righteous, and when it is not? Imagine the Christian who is diagnosed with a terminal illness, and her only treatment option is an experimental drug that is costly, has potentially dangerous side effects, and has a low probability of success. Is she obligated to pursue this treatment, or is refusing the treatment and accepting death a morally righteous choice? Or what about the Christian who can survive only by undergoing dialysis very frequently and is unable to live a normal and productive life? Must he continue dialysis under every condition, or does there come a point when he could ethically decide to forgo it? What are Christians to do if they are compelled to care for a relative who has entered a persistent vegetative state (PVS), the condition of now famous figures like Karen Ann Quinlan, Nancy Cruzan, and Terri Schiavo? Should they provide artificial nutrition and hydration (ANH) to such a patient, or is letting her die the morally sound decision?

Many readers have already had to make decisions like these for themselves or their loved ones, or have been asked to assist others who have had to make such decisions. Readers who have not faced such a situation will likely do so in the future. Modern medical technology has not eliminated death, but it has developed great capabilities to delay it and to preserve people in conditions that previous generations would not have imagined. How can Christians make godly decisions when many of the questions are so new and the Bible offers little specific guidance?

In my experience there are many Christians who assume that because they are "pro-life" they are obligated to extend life as long as possible. Yet often such Christians also sense that seeking to extend life indefinitely creates terrible situations that they wish to avoid— but feel guilty for having such thoughts. On the other hand, there are also many Christians who readily succumb to the patterns of worldly thinking that assert that people are free to choose death at any time for the sake of avoiding pain or inconvenience. In my judgment, fidelity to the Christian moral life means neither assuming that life should always be extended as long as possible nor assuming that death can be chosen anytime that life seems burdensome. The claims of Christian truth challenge both worldly exaltation of human choice and overly simplistic notions of what it means to be "pro-life." As we explore the implications of Christian truth for decisions about accepting and forgoing treatment, it is important to keep in mind that there are many cases for which there are no clear-cut, black-and-white answers. We are delving into areas where Scripture has provided little explicit instruction to bind the conscience of Christians. Thus Christians must seek to exercise godly wisdom and discernment as they make these judgments upon which life and death depend. We should not expect to determine right and wrong answers simply by plugging data into the right ethical formulas. Each of us must make his own decisions, after seeking wise counsel from others, and not impose our particular judgments upon the conscience of others, who must exercise their own God-given wisdom.

We will first consider some common categories that bioethics writers use to resolve questions about accepting and refusing treatment. Then we will consider a number of basic guidelines, derived from the truths of Christian theology, that should help us to make godly decisions. Finally we will look at several concrete scenarios and explore how to put the basic guidelines into practice in these difficult situations.

Common Categories

To begin, it may be helpful to identify and to evaluate a few common categories that other writers use to resolve these ethical problems. One common category that appears in discussions of accepting and forgoing medical care is the distinction between *ordinary* and *extraordinary* treatment. This distinction usually identifies ordinary treatment as that which a person is obligated to accept and extraordinary treatment as that which a person has liberty to refuse. For this distinction to be useful, criteria for determining what is ordinary and what is extraordinary must be established. Perhaps unsurprisingly, writers who employ this distinction have failed to come to consensus about what these criteria are. Is it the nature of the treatment itself that distinguishes ordinary from extraordinary? In other words, is ordinary treatment that which is routine, simple, or inexpensive (such as taking penicillin) and extraordinary treatment that which is experimental, difficult to endure, or very costly? Or, as some authors have argued, should the distinction pertain not simply to the treatment itself but to the whole circumstances surrounding the patient who is considering the treatment, such that what is ordinary for one patient may be extraordinary for another? Because I believe that this distinction is inherently ambiguous, I do not employ it in this chapter. Nevertheless, both the character of the treatment and the holistic circumstances of the patient are of moral relevance for end-of-life ethical questions (as I discuss below).

Another common category, especially in Roman Catholic literature, is the principle of *double effect*. This idea, which is also applied in other areas of ethics, states that it may be permissible to perform an action that produces an evil effect if the primary intent of the action is to bring about a different effect that is good. This principle also requires that the evil effect not be the means for accomplishing the good effect and that the good which is accomplished outweighs the evil proportionally. For example, it may be permissible to administer an analgesic to a dying patient even though that may hasten the onset of death. Hastening death is an evil effect, according to this analysis, but the primary intent is the good effect of reducing the patient's pain. The evil effect is a foreseen, though not intended, consequence. In my judgment, the basic insight behind the principle of double effect is correct. A person's intention can have moral significance and, in a fallen world, it is sometimes proper to pursue certain goods even when we foresee that evil may also result. I am not persuaded, however, that the traditional Roman Catholic criteria for applying this principle are always helpful or that they must determine the application of the principle on every occasion. Thus I do not employ this category as such.

Finally, some people make a distinction between *withholding* and *withdrawing* treatment. The distinction itself is easy to understand. Withholding treatment refers to the decision not to begin a certain kind of medical care in the first place, while withdrawing treatment refers to the decision to stop a certain kind of medical care that is presently being administered. Those who employ this distinction usually mean to suggest that there are circumstances when it is morally permissible to withhold treatment in the first place but that once treatment has begun it is not permissible to withdraw it. According to this train of thought, initiating treatment creates certain expectations and commitments that produce more stringent moral criteria for justifying its subsequent discontinuation. In my judgment, the proposed distinction between withholding and withdrawing treatment is not morally significant, and it is not possible to identify different sets of criteria for evaluating each one. As some writers have noted, insisting upon the moral significance of this distinction may have the unintended negative effect of discouraging people from beginning useful treatments, because they fear that they will be bound to a course of treatment that they will not be able to refuse at a later date. Accordingly, in this chapter I ordinarily use the word "forgo" as a general term that includes both "withholding" and "withdrawing."

The Significance of Intention

We can now consider some basic guidelines for decisions about accepting and forgoing treatment. The first matter for consideration regards *intention*. When discussing the principle of double effect, I noted my belief that intention is a morally significant aspect of decisions to forgo treatment. In part, I made this point in chapter 8, where I argued for the distinction between killing and letting die and claimed that decisions to stop fighting the threat of death may be not a choice to die but rather a choice for a certain kind of life (albeit a shorter one). Of course, intention is not the only significant factor. Having a good intention does not justify an inherently evil act. But when faced with choices that cannot be labeled inherently good or evil, the intentions and motivations behind the choice are morally relevant.

Two brief considerations help to explain this conclusion. First, Scripture itself makes crucial moral distinctions based upon a person's intention. For example, the Mosaic law often distinguishes between those who kill intentionally and those who do not (e.g., Ex. 21:12–14; Num. 35:9–34; Deut. 19:13). The Mosaic law even establishes cities of refuge for those who kill unintentionally and seek protection from those who might take vengeance upon them: "If anyone kills his neighbor unintentionally without having hated him in the past—as when someone goes into the forest with his neighbor to cut wood, and his hand swings the axe to cut down a tree, and the head slips from the handle and strikes his neighbor so that he dies—he may flee to one of these cities and live" (Deut. 19:4–5). These cities of refuge served special purposes for Old Testament Israel, but there is nothing unique about the distinction between those who kill willfully and those who do not. Contemporary American law makes the same distinction. It even has a middle category referred to as manslaughter, covering cases in which a killer did not intend to kill and thus is not guilty of murder, but acted recklessly when he killed and thus is held accountable on a lesser charge. As a general legal matter, therefore, people judge the same external act in radically different ways depending upon the intent of the actor.

Second, the importance of virtue for a holistic understanding of the moral life highlights the significance of intention. God has called believers not simply to perform certain sorts of actions but also to be a certain kind of people. These two aspects of the moral life—what we do and what sort of character we have—are inseparable. It is precisely virtuous people who perform righteous actions and right-acting people who grow in virtue. In light of this, a holistic moral account of decisions about forgoing treatment must pay attention not only to external actions but also to the kind of person who performs these actions. Are a person's actions flowing out of God-honoring virtues? To answer this question we must know *why* a person is choosing a course of action and *what goals* she is seeking to achieve.

These considerations mean that we must ask *why* we make the choices that we make about accepting and forgoing medical treatment. Am I choosing to forgo treatment because I am aiming to achieve death, that is, because death is my goal? If so, then the decision is morally problematic. Christians must refuse to seek death, whether for ourselves or for others. Or, am I choosing to forgo treatment not in order to die but in order to live a certain kind of life that the treatment would make impossible? If so, then the decision may be a godly one. Our intentions are closely linked to the virtues. For example, is someone's decision to forgo a burdensome course of chemotherapy that offers only a remote chance of a cure the product of courage (which emboldens him to face death) or of hope (which draws his eyes away from the disappointments of this life)? Or is this decision the product of cowardice (which shrinks before fear of the discomfort of chemotherapy) or of despair (which tempts him to give up on life)? When the choice flows from virtue, we can have greater confidence that it is morally sound than when it flows from vice.

In real life, of course, we usually act with mixed motives and conflicting intentions, and this especially so when the decisions are particularly complicated and life-shaping. No one should be deceived into thinking that discerning his intentions is easy. "The purpose in a man's heart is like deep water, but a man of understanding will draw it out" (Prov. 20:5). This biblical proverb not only reminds us of the difficulty of sifting through the conflicting intentions of a sinful heart, but also encourages us that this task is not impossible. What is required for the task is *understanding*. In other words, the person who is wise according to the teaching of Proverbs—being virtuous, discerning, and morally mature—will be in a much better position to make difficult decisions about accepting and forgoing treatment than one who is not wise. This is a reminder, then, that making end-of-life decisions is not simply a matter of memorizing a series of rules. Each individual must strive through the whole of life to become the kind of virtuous and wise person who is prepared to make these difficult choices.

Treatment Decisions and Human Goods

In establishing guidelines for accepting and forgoing treatment, it is also necessary to investigate the goods or ends that we intend to achieve through our choices. God made us not simply to follow rules but to achieve worthy goals. When Christians are wrestling with ethical problems for which there is no clear biblical rule, therefore, it is important that they identify which goals are in fact worthy of pursuit. We should not slip into patterns of earthly thinking and shape our conduct for the purpose of attaining selfish ends. Instead, we should strive to achieve ends that are God-honoring and promote true human flourishing for ourselves and others. I refer to such ends as "good ends" or simply "goods."

The preservation of life is a good end, and thus the decision to accept medical treatment is ordinarily a righteous choice. But the preservation of life is not the *only* good end, which is precisely why the issues addressed in this chapter can be so difficult. As Christians we should not single-mindedly aim to make life as long as possible, but should strive to live fruitful and beneficial lives for however many days God gives us. In other words, we should aim to live the right *kind* of life, not necessarily the *longest* life. Sometimes in fact the choice to live the right kind of life means that we cannot choose to live as long as possible. No single action can ever attain all the good ends that God has placed before human beings, and in particular situations we must choose which goods we will seek to attain and which we will not. Sometimes in choosing to forgo treatment, and thereby hastening death, we seek to attain good ends distinct from the good of preserving life.

Our task here is to identify other goods *in addition to the preservation of life* that may be relevant to decisions about forgoing treatment. It is important to remember that simply because we can identify another valuable good that might be achieved by forgoing treatment does not mean that forgoing treatment is necessarily the best decision. The whole situation, with all of the possible goods that are at stake, must be taken into account if a person is to make a morally responsible choice.

Spiritual Goods

The most important good ends that are often relevant for difficult end-of-life decisions are spiritual goods. Our religious devotion and obedient allegiance to God must always be our first priority. As the Lord Jesus said, "Seek first the kingdom of God and his righteousness, and all these things will be added to you" (Matt. 6:33). The various earthly goods concerning our own physical health and welfare must take a backseat to pursuing the good of God's kingdom and his righteousness (Matt. 6:25–32). Earlier in the Sermon on the Mount Jesus makes a similar point and puts it in even starker terms: "If your right eye causes you to sin, tear it out and throw it away. For it is better that you lose one of your members than that your whole body be thrown into hell. And if your right hand causes you to sin, cut if off and throw it away. For it is better that you lose one of your members than that your whole body go into hell" (Matt. 5:29–30). His manner of speaking is certainly hyperbolic, for he does not promote literal self-mutilation. But Jesus' broader point is crucial for the present discussion. Even the wholeness and integrity of our physical bodies are less important than pursuing the righteousness and holiness that Jesus proclaims in this Sermon. Our spiritual integrity is of higher value than our physical integrity, and though the latter is a good worth pursuing, the former takes priority when we must choose between them. The most extreme application of this is the case of martyrdom. Christians ought not to seek to be killed for the sake of Christ, but when forsaking Christ is the price of preserving life, the Christian must choose allegiance to Christ.

What does this have to do with bioethics? Christians ought to consider how their choices about accepting and forgoing treatment will bear upon the pursuit of their spiritual welfare and religious devotion. It is difficult to explore this in the abstract, so pondering a concrete case may illustrate. Our religious devotion includes the obligations to gather with God's people in worship on the Lord's Day (e.g., see Ex. 20:8–11; Acts 20:7; Heb. 10:24–25) and to pray continually (1 Thess. 5:17). These are not absolute commands, in that illness and disability can make these tasks temporarily impossible. But prayer, hearing the Word preached, and receiving the sacraments are crucial requirements for our growth in grace, and we must pursue them actively. Ordinarily, caring for our bodies and receiving medical treatment promote our health and thus make us better able to avail ourselves of these blessings. But sometimes this is not the case. If a course of medical treatment threatens to hinder our religious devotion—for example, by incapacitating us and thus prohibiting attendance at worship services, or by dulling our minds and hence keeping us from prayer—but does not offer any long-term promise of promoting our religious devotion, then forgoing such treatment may be the righteous decision for the Christian.

Earthly Goods

In addition to spiritual goods and the preservation of life, various earthly goods can be worth pursuing when we face end-of-life treatment decisions. Among these earthly goods are physical comfort, the fellowship of family and friends, and the ability to work and play. Of course we should not pursue these things in a way that is self-centered or harmful to others. Sometimes we must give up such things in order to promote other people's welfare or to remain loyal to Christ. In and of themselves, however, these things are truly *goods*. God made us in his image to be social and hard-working creatures who enjoy the abundance of this earth. Pursuing these earthly goods is thus morally upright.

The relevant question is whether a proposed course of treatment would aid us in achieving these valuable human goods. This line of inquiry raises questions about "quality of life." This is a slippery phrase that different people use in different ways. Some people use the idea of "quality of life" to ask whether certain sorts of lives are no longer valuable or not worth living. For example, suppose that a course of treatment would prevent me from dying but result in a poor quality of life, because it would lead to physical discomfort and prevent me from performing many activities that I enjoy. Should I forgo treatment because I would be better off dead than experiencing such a life? I suggest that this is a morally problematic use of the "quality of life" idea. All human life is valuable and, as discussed in chapter 8, it is never our prerogative to seek death because of despair and discouragement. There is a better use of the "quality of life" idea, however. It is proper to ask whether life without treatment or life with treatment would be *better*. The question is not about choosing life or death, but about choosing which sort of life (though we know that one choice might bring death sooner). This question is therefore similar to the one that I posed in regard to spiritual goods: will this treatment benefit or hinder my pursuit of valuable earthly goods?

One specific consideration that helps to answer this question is the extent of suffering that *the treatment itself* would bring. We should not inflict death upon ourselves, and likewise we should not, in general, inflict lesser bodily harms and physical discomforts upon ourselves. Inflicting pain upon ourselves for its own sake—masochism—is morally perverted. Under ordinary circumstances we do not allow people to inject poison into our veins or to cut open our abdomens, and avoiding such procedures is a good worthy of pursuit. At times we submit ourselves to chemotherapy or surgery, but only because we judge that the suffering will be outweighed by a greater good, such as the restoration of health or the preservation of life itself. The fact that we reason in this way indicates that, when we are deciding whether to accept or to forgo treatment, the degree of suffering it will produce is a morally relevant factor. I might judge that a shorter life free from the suffering produced by that treatment is better than a longer life that must endure that suffering.

Another specific consideration involves the kind of life that a person would lead *as a result of the treatment* (assuming that the treatment is successful). Again I remind the reader that I am not raising this issue as if to suggest that we might simply decide to die because we judge that our life would no longer be worth living. Many treatments offer promise of success only at the cost of significant suffering on the other end. Some treatments, even if successful, will leave us incapacitated and unable to pursue normal, productive activities and unable to enjoy ordinary interaction with other people. This fact raises questions about my general obligation as an image bearer of God to foster the capacity to work and to cultivate opportunities for relationships with fellow human beings. Ordinarily we ought not to do things or to allow other people to do things to us that hinder or prohibit such activities, though there are particular circumstances when other valuable goods will outweigh this general moral principle and thus compel us to choose differently. The fact that we reason in this way indicates that the kind of life that awaits us on the other side of treatment is a relevant consideration when faced with the choice between accepting and forgoing that treatment. A Christian might decide that a (shorter) life without the treatment is better than a (longer) life that results from the treatment, because the former permits us to pursue certain image-bearing tasks (though perhaps only briefly) that the latter does not.

A third specific consideration is the effect that a proposed course of treatment would have upon other people. This consideration also must be handled with care. I am not suggesting that a person should try to evaluate the worth of her life over against the worth of other people's lives (or their time or money). But since our creation in the image of God makes us social creatures with mutual responsibilities, and since love for our neighbor is a primary Christian virtue, the good of others is a valuable end that each of us ought to pursue. I should not make treatment decisions for myself without considering others. One person's choice to accept or forgo treatment usually impinges upon other people's lives, sometimes in drastic and life-shaping ways.

When we face a treatment decision, therefore, we should consider whether accepting or forgoing treatment would better foster our relationship with others and promote their flourishing.

Ordinarily accepting treatment will be the better choice. If treatment extends my life and restores my health, then I am able to continue loving and being a blessing to other people, whereas refusing such treatment and succumbing to death would bring great suffering upon my loved ones. But forgoing treatment may seem the better choice in some situations. In certain cases forgoing treatment will permit interaction and activities with loved ones, even for a brief time, that accepting the treatment will permanently prohibit, even if it succeeds in prolonging life. In other cases accepting treatment will place onerous burdens upon other people, such as crushing financial liabilities. To raise such matters treads on delicate ground, for we cannot put a monetary value on a human life. Yet it is a fact that we live in a world of scarcity. Ideally the cost of my medical treatment would not matter, for human life is more valuable than money. But resources are limited and no individual, family, or society can spend all of its assets and energy on medical care. In the United States and many other first world countries the rising cost of health care is a major social issue. Medical costs strain government budgets and bankrupt families. As difficult as such decisions can be, there come times when a person must ask whether it is morally responsible to pursue a course of treatment that will bring financial ruin or other major disruption upon his family. Of course it is a good thing for people to make great financial sacrifices for loved ones who are gravely ill. Loving self-sacrifice should work in both directions, however. If I am gravely ill, surely there are times when an expensive treatment will bring little enough benefit to my health or life expectancy that to insist upon receiving it would be a violation of the obligation to love my family and to seek their prosperity rather than impoverishment.

On a related note, it may also be proper in some cases for a person to ask which sort of life—life with treatment or life without it—will likely lead to the kind of death that is relatively more edifying and relatively less tragic for his family and friends. In all of these situations we should never choose death over life, but morally responsible people should reflect upon whether life without treatment (though it may be short) or life with treatment will do more to promote the flourishing of other people.

Choosing among These Human Goods

To this point I have identified several valuable goods that Christians should consider as they ponder decisions about accepting or forgoing medical treatment. There is no mathematical formula that will yield a clear moral answer if we simply plug in the particular goods that may be at stake in a particular situation. We must constantly pursue a range of goods, yet seldom can we pursue all of them simultaneously, and often we must deliberately choose to pursue one of them and not another. We should never choose to do something that is evil in itself (such as committing suicide), but how we decide which goods to pursue in a given situation is a matter of judgment and discretion. Before turning to discuss some particular scenarios, let us examine a couple considerations that may be of help for making these discretionary judgments about medical treatment.

The first consideration concerns the likelihood that a treatment will be successful. Earlier I argued that it is morally responsible to ask whether the life we would live after treatment *if it is successful* is a better life than the one we would live if we were to forgo treatment. But of course treatments sometimes fail. An inherent unpredictability plagues all human endeavors, but this is especially evident in medical procedures. No treatment has a 100 percent success rate. Treatments range from having very high to very low probabilities of success. Many kinds of treatments are so new and experimental that the likelihood of success is impossible to predict. We cannot be certain whether a treatment will produce the effects that it promises, but what we do know about the likelihood of a treatment's success ought to influence our moral judgments. For example, suppose that someone is weighing whether to accept treatment that promises to restore him to a fair state of health, but which will certainly make him feel miserable while he receives it. In this case the probability of the treatment's success is clearly relevant for his decision whether to endure this miserable treatment for the sake of recovering his health. What he would be willing to endure for the sake of a 95 percent chance of recovery is probably not what he would be willing to endure for the sake of a 5 percent chance of recovery. As a side note, I suggest that this consideration should encourage us all the more to solicit the best medical advice that we are able to attain, in order to acquire a sense of how likely a successful outcome is. Physicians sometimes have incentive to keep their patients from knowing how unlikely it is that a course of treatment will be successful, so patients are wise to ask pointed questions about such things.

The second consideration is the patient's stage of life when she is choosing whether to accept or to forgo treatment. In exploring this idea Daniel Callahan has argued that death should be seen as a part of life, giving shape to life's trajectory and meaningfulness. Since death is an integral part of life and is its natural end, writes Callahan, a person can view his death as acceptable, and not premature or tragic, if most of his capacities for selfhood have been lost and further attempts to preserve life are liable to deform the dying process. Callahan's reasoning indicates that a person should be more apt to forgo treatments when he has reached the stage of life when death is acceptable and natural and should be more apt to accept treatments when he retains many capacities for exercising human personhood, such that death would be tragic and premature. Callahan's reasoning is humane and generally seems to yield sensible judgments about end-of-life treatment decisions. One thing that should give readers pause, however, is that Callahan contrasts his position with that of certain Christian theologians who do not view death as natural or acceptable, but as an enemy and the ultimate insult. Callahan winsomely sets these two different perspectives on death in front of his readers. How should we respond to this choice?

From a Christian theological standpoint, Callahan's perspective on death is fundamentally flawed. Though Christians have been released from the curse of death through the work of Christ, death has not therefore become natural. Death is inherently unnatural, contrary to the original order of creation. In my judgment, nevertheless, the stage of life in which a person faces a momentous treatment decision is indeed relevant, and aspects of Callahan's discussion remain helpful. Even within the confines of the fallen world, God has established a regular order of things. After the flood God promised to preserve the natural order: "While the earth remains, seedtime and harvest, cold and heat, summer and winter, day and night, shall not cease" (Gen. 8:22). This regularity of nature extends also to the span of human life. Before the flood God declared: "My Spirit shall not abide in man forever, for he is flesh: his days shall be 120 years" (Gen. 6:3). Later the psalmist reflected upon the course and brevity of human life and noted that the "years of our life are seventy, or even by reason of strength eighty . . ." (Ps. 90:10). Today, after so many generations and the advance of medical technology, these biblical statements about the boundaries of human life are still remarkably accurate. Seventy to eighty years remain for us an ordinary span of life, and the upper limit in cases of extremely long life is about 120 years. Thus there is an ordinary length for human life, and this fact makes "life expectancy" a reasonable idea. We instinctively understand that a person who fails to reach seventy or eighty years has died, by ordinary human standards, prematurely. We instinctively judge that a child's death at age nine is a tragedy in a way that an elderly person's death at age ninety-nine is not. Death is our enemy—this is a profound theological truth that Christians must affirm. But death is also ordinary and natural at certain stages of life and not others, when viewed in terms of the divinely established boundaries of this fallen yet preserved world.

What does this mean, then, for decisions about accepting and forgoing treatment? I suggest that it plays a helpful role in concrete situations when we must evaluate and compare the various goods identified earlier. Someone weighing whether a (shorter) life without a course of treatment may be better than a (longer) life with it has many relevant considerations to ponder. Among these relevant considerations are how much longer that longer life would likely be and what sorts of human goods she could reasonably expect to pursue with that longer life. For both of these considerations her stage of life is crucially relevant information. A person at an advanced stage of life cannot expect a significantly longer life even with treatment. Nor can she expect, even under the best of circumstances, to be able to pursue the range of human goods that a younger person could. Again it is important to offer caution that there are no clear-cut, black-and-white lines here. It is not as if people who are below a certain age should accept treatments and those who are above that age should forgo them. But when we must make difficult decisions about treatments and therefore must choose one way of life over another, the stage of life in which we find ourselves must affect our moral reasoning.

Particular Scenarios

In the light of these guidelines for decisions about accepting or forgoing treatment, let us consider some particular scenarios and explore how to apply these guidelines with wisdom. Space permits discussion of only a few potential situations. Many difficult treatment decisions, however, will resemble cases like the four that I identify and discuss.

What is more important than being able to slot our own situation into a pre-identified case with a ready-made answer is growing in our ability to think in a morally mature and God-pleasing way about whatever complex, tragic, and troubling situation we may face.

The Otherwise Terminal Illness That Is Curable with a Long-Shot Treatment

The first sort of scenario is this: a person has a life-threatening illness, and the available treatment offers only a remote chance of recovery. Such a scenario may arise when an experimental drug or procedure is being developed, perhaps to fight a deadly cancer or to provide a transplant. As a concrete example, we might imagine a woman in her thirties fighting leukemia. She has been brought into remission after relapse but she is certain to face another relapse and then death if she does not receive a bone marrow transplant. Yet her physicians have been unable to find a suitable adult marrow donor, and the only available course of treatment is an experimental transplant using umbilical cord stem cells. Because of the many uncertainties surrounding this experimental procedure, her physicians have indicated that it has only a 20 percent chance of success. How should she and her family decide whether to pursue this treatment?

The incentive for pursuing the procedure is obvious. Every expectation points to death in the near future if she forgoes treatment, while the treatment holds out the possibility of survival and cure from her leukemia. A possible answer is that treatment should certainly be pursued, because even an 80 percent chance of death is better than a 100 percent chance. In light of the considerations raised earlier, however, a number of factors suggest that life without this transplant (though possibly shorter) might be better than life with the transplant (though possibly longer). One factor is that the treatment itself would entail a great deal of suffering, if not in the stem-cell transplant itself at least in the full-body radiation and intensive chemotherapy before the transplant and the long recovery afterward. This recovery would likely involve graft-versus-host disease and frequent transfusions while her blood counts are recovering. Furthermore, a very unpleasant kind of death via graft-versus-host disease could well follow the transplant. These factors offer compelling reasons why she might conclude that life without the treatment would likely be better than the life she could expect to face with the treatment. Without the transplant she would live for some time feeling relatively well and leading a fairly normal life, and then, following the inevitable relapse, would die a gradual and relatively painless death from the leukemia. With the transplant, on the other hand, she would immediately subject herself to great hardship, make an unpleasant death relatively likely, and, if the transplant goes poorly from the start, perhaps even die sooner than if the transplant had never occurred.

Added to this are many uncertainties about the consequences of the transplant, even if it is successful in curing the leukemia. For example, what sort of damage might her internal organs suffer as side effects of the radiation and chemotherapy required before the transplant? Would these side effects prevent her from living a normal life even if she survives the transplant, and how sharply would they lower her life expectancy? Furthermore, even if she has good insurance coverage, her family is likely to sustain considerable personal and financial costs in their efforts to care for her properly. She could reasonably conclude that it would be better to forgo the transplant and enjoy a short but wholesome time with loved ones than to undergo the transplant with its attendant trials and sufferings.

In light of these things, a morally responsible argument can be made in favor of forgoing the treatment and choosing a possibly shorter but better life, with its prospects for quality time with family and friends and then for a painless and peaceful death. Yet the possibility, however small, of regaining a relatively normal life is a strongly attractive prospect that is not easily outweighed. Many circumstances of this woman's life were left unstated above. Is she the mother of young children who would be especially harmed by her death? What other familial or community responsibilities does she have? Is she in the midst of a meaningful project to which she has devoted years of her life but has not yet finished? All of these factors might drive her (though would not require her) to pursue the treatment in spite of the many hardships that the transplant would bring upon her and her loved ones. As she decides upon a course of action, she should strive for courage to do what she judges right, and strive not to be swayed by a cowardly fear of death or of the transplant. She should also undertake her decision with contentment toward God in light of all of his blessings, despite the tragic circumstances in which she finds herself.

The Chronic Illness with a Burdensome Treatment

The next specific scenario concerns a person who has a chronic illness that medical treatment can contain but cannot cure. For some serious and otherwise fatal illnesses medical treatment can keep a person alive with some degree of functionality, but the treatment itself lays a great burden upon him. An example of this is a middle-aged man with kidney failure who is not able to procure a kidney transplant. Frequent and lengthy dialysis sessions keep him alive, though in a weakened state unable to perform many of life's basic activities. In such a state he wonders whether discontinuing dialysis and accepting imminent death would be a morally legitimate decision. How should we evaluate this sort of situation?

This scenario has certain similarities to the transplant case, as well as significant differences. Like the previous case, this patient has an ailment that will kill him if left untreated. But unlike the previous case, the treatment itself offers high probability of success yet offers no probability of a cure. Another difference is that while the leukemia patient would likely be able to live a relatively normal life for a short time if she refuses treatment, this dialysis patient would certainly live for only a very brief time after stopping dialysis, and even in that brief time he would not enjoy normal human activity. These differences, I believe, make a decision to forgo treatment in the present case more difficult to defend than in the previous case. One important reason why it is more difficult to defend is that this patient does not seem to have genuine *life* choices before him. Unlike the transplant patient, who has a choice between a short but productive life and a possibly longer but suffering-filled life, this dialysis patient's choice is between an imminent death and indefinitely prolonged suffering. Forgoing dialysis will give him no window in which he can build a treehouse for his grandchildren or visit a cousin across the country. The choice to forgo seems to be a choice to die rather than to live. As considered in chapter 8, the believer ought not to choose death as an end. Those who live suffering-filled lives deserve all of our love and compassion, but the fact that someone really does not like his life does not give him justification to end it. We may seek to improve the life that we have, but we are also called to endure the hardships of life that we cannot change. Christians are called to suffer piously, in union with the Christ who suffered before them. Life with dialysis may not be as rich and productive as life without the need for dialysis. But if a

Christian finds himself in this situation, then as far as possible he
should seek new goods to pursue even with his limited capacities. By
faith he must trust that the Lord will bless that pursuit, for himself
and for others, though he may struggle to understand how that will
happen.

Insofar as the choice to stop dialysis is a decision to die because of
the hardship of life, therefore, it is morally problematic. The question that remains is this: can a decision to stop dialysis be something
other than a choice to die? I believe that the answer is affirmative.
One of the valuable human goods is the absence of pain and suffering. Generally speaking, it is morally deviant for a person to
inflict such things upon himself willingly. Thus one of the morally
relevant considerations for making a treatment decision is the extent
of suffering that the *treatment itself* inflicts. Though the restoration
of health or the preservation of life ordinarily makes the decision
to undergo burdensome treatment a good choice, there obviously
must come a point at which a course of treatment itself inflicts so
much suffering that the choice to avoid it is morally sound. We
must strive for courage in the midst of hardship, but we are not
called to torture ourselves. Though dialysis is presumably never the
equivalent of torture in terms of physical pain, it is conceivable that
the whole package of physical, spiritual, and emotional burdens of
regular dialysis treatment could amount to an unbearable burden
for a person. In such a case, the decision to forgo further treatment
need not be judged as a choice of death over life, but rather as a
choice to avoid an imposition of unbearable burden, though death
will be the tragic consequence.

Another occasion in which a decision to forgo dialysis might be a
morally righteous decision is when the patient has a terminal illness
in addition to the kidney failure and is approaching death because of
that terminal illness. If continuing dialysis is simply staving off death
from kidney failure in order to die imminently from something else,
there is no compelling reason to insist that dialysis must go on. In
this situation the choice is not even between death and life—it is
between one kind of death and another kind of death. The Christian
may rightly choose to succumb to the affliction that provides the
best opportunity to die in spiritual communion with the Lord and in
fellowship with loved ones. A different analysis is necessary, however,
if death from the terminal illness is not in fact imminent. A terminal

diagnosis does not necessarily mean imminent death. In a situation in which a person could expect to live with his terminal illness for a substantial period of time and to pursue meaningful human activities, forgoing dialysis and succumbing to an imminent death from kidney failure would seem to be more a choice of death over life than a choice between two different kinds of life.

Treatment for the Terminal Patient

The last scenario prompts consideration of another sort of scenario. How should a patient diagnosed with a terminal illness make decisions about treatments designed to prolong her life, though there is no hope for a cure or even for an indefinite extension of life? This scenario is different from that of the dialysis patient for whom dialysis would extend life indefinitely. In the present scenario the patient is going to die imminently. A concrete example is a woman who has been diagnosed with a cancer that cannot be cured through present medical technology. How should she decide whether to continue chemotherapy treatments that cannot cure but only stave off death for a little longer, or whether to receive pain medications that may hasten death?

These questions take us back to a key question raised in the preceding case: is she choosing between two different kinds of life, or is she choosing between life and death? And if she is genuinely choosing between two different kinds of life, what are the valuable human goods at stake in each of the two choices? It is probably the case that the choice about additional chemotherapy is indeed between two kinds of life, a shorter one without treatment and a somewhat longer one with treatment. The factors that could sway the decision are the degree of burdensomeness of the chemotherapy, the length of time she could expect the chemotherapy to extend her life, and the kinds of meaningful activities that she could pursue with and without the chemotherapy. If the chemotherapy itself would produce great hardship, constrain meaningful interaction with loved ones, and offer only a brief respite from death, then the decision to forgo chemotherapy is probably the better choice. On the other hand, if the chemotherapy would not be overly burdensome, would enhance rather than reduce meaningful interaction with loved ones, and would offer more than a minimal extension of life expectancy, then the better decision is probably to accept the treatment.

Is it morally justified, furthermore, to accept pain medication that not only relieves her physical discomfort but also might hasten death? As a general matter there is no moral objection to using analgesics. Since pain is one of the great curses brought by illness, the ability of modern medicine to reduce pain significantly in nearly every situation is a great technological achievement. In situations where death-hastening doses of analgesics are necessary in order to keep a terminal cancer patient in relative comfort, death is probably near anyway. Under such conditions, the choice whether to act in a way that may hasten an already imminent death seems to be a choice between two (very short) kinds of life. If one sort of life (and death) involves great pain and the other does not, the choice to accept the pain medication seems morally sound.

The Persistent Vegetative State

The final scenario to be considered is the persistent vegetative state (PVS), one of the most hotly discussed topics in end-of-life care. PVS patients are in a condition of permanent unconsciousness due to a total loss of higher-brain functions. They have no awareness of themselves or their environment and no sensation of pain. But because their brain stems continue to function, they breathe spontaneously, open their eyes, and have sleep-wake cycles. Since swallowing is a voluntary action, PVS patients can only survive through provision of artificial nutrition and hydration (ANH), through a feeding tube of some form. PVS patients do not necessarily have any other medical ailment, thus they often live for extended periods of time if ANH is provided. In light of their potentially long life expectancy in a state of complete unresponsiveness and unconsciousness, the question of how to treat such patients has understandably been difficult and controversial. Few writers dispute that it is permissible and humane for the PVS patient's proxy to decide that he should not receive seriously invasive procedures, such as coronary bypass surgery. But writers have registered serious disagreements about whether proxies may decline ANH for the patient. Most writers conclude that this is a morally sound choice, though some Christian writers, both Protestant and Roman Catholic, argue that it is not. Being in a PVS state is a rare condition, but it presents a challenging ethical scenario and serves as an interesting test for the moral guidelines presented earlier.

Some have argued in favor of forgoing ANH for PVS patients on the ground that these patients should be considered dead already. Proponents of this idea reject the commonly accepted "whole-brain" definition of death and believe that those who have permanently lost their higher-brain functions should be declared dead even if brain stem functions continue. This idea corresponds to an understanding of human personhood commonly described as "functional" or "biographical," in distinction from "essential" or "biological," as discussed in chapter 5. Though undertaking a range of human activities in relationship with others is an important aspect of the image of God, personhood cannot be reduced to such things, and thus the functional or biographical definition should be rejected. The capability of modern medical technology to preserve various bodily functions has indeed made it difficult in some situations to define precisely when death occurs. But Christian theology reminds us that the image of God does not reside only in the human soul in distinction from the body. Scripture generally regards death as the separation of soul and body (e.g., Matt. 27:50; Acts 20:10), but we have no empirical way to determine the exact point when that separation takes place. Since a living human person, an image bearer of God, is both soul *and* body united, the continuing functioning of the body is compelling evidence that the soul is still present and that a person is not dead. It is pertinent to recall that the PVS patient sleeps and wakes, opens and closes his eyes, and gags and coughs. This patient's body operates normally in many respects. It is also pertinent to recall the way in which Ecclesiastes 12:7 describes death, as the body's return to the earth and the spirit's return to God. The PVS patient's body is not decaying and thus is not returning to the dust of the ground. In light of these considerations, I conclude that we should not consider the PVS patient dead. The question about ANH cannot be brushed aside so easily.

Most people who argue that it is morally acceptable to forgo ANH for a PVS patient operate on the assumption that the patient is still alive. Sometimes they appeal to notions of mercy or death with dignity. For reasons that we considered when discussing physician-assisted suicide and euthanasia, I do not believe that such appeals are morally persuasive, at least if they stand alone. What then are the key moral questions for Christians who wish to make decisions for PVS patients that are consistent with the moral guidelines suggested earlier?

One important question that has been raised is whether providing ANH for PVS patients constitutes basic care or medical treatment. This is a significant question because of the basic moral axiom that though caregivers may discontinue medical treatment in certain circumstances, they must always provide basic care. This is illustrated by the case of the patient with terminal cancer considered previously. Caregivers are morally obligated to continue to feed, clothe, and bathe her as she approaches death, even after they have discontinued chemotherapy. Along these lines, some opponents of forgoing ANH for PVS patients argue that ANH is basic care, not medical treatment, because the need for nutrition and hydration is a universal human need, not a fatal illness. The PVS patient has no underlying terminal condition and therefore is not dying. To withhold ANH from a PVS patient is killing him by starvation/dehydration, not simply allowing him to die from a fatal malady. Thus, while forgoing a kidney transplant for a PVS patient is morally acceptable, forgoing ANH is fundamentally different and constitutes a failure of our most basic obligations toward a helpless patient.

This line of argument is compelling in many ways, but there are also strong counterarguments. For one thing, though providing food and drink to patients under ordinary conditions is basic care rather than medical treatment, installing a feeding tube and maintaining it when complications arise are medical procedures that require the work of a physician, not basic care that can simply be entrusted to nurses. Furthermore, though the PVS patient may not suffer from a terminal illness in the same sense that a person with an advanced case of cancer does, he does have an underlying pathology that prevents him from eating and drinking and that would bring about his death in relatively short order, apart from modern medical technology. Building on this point, some writers have noted that use of the term "starvation" portrays the situation in misleading ways. For one thing, "starvation" ordinarily indicates a death that is painful and unpleasant, but the PVS patient experiences nothing of the sort. Second, apart from the PVS context, it is common for a person approaching the end of life to lose his appetite and to cease eating, a situation that we would not term "starvation." This loss of appetite and refusal of food may in fact hasten death, but often does so in merciful, not hardship producing, ways.

This "basic care" versus "medical treatment" debate is not easy to mediate, and it is actually compelling to conclude that the provision of ANH for a PVS patient is *both* basic care *and* medical treatment. The need for nutrition and hydration cannot be considered a terminal ailment, otherwise everybody on the planet should be reckoned as terminal and the concept becomes meaningless. Therefore providing ANH for a PVS patient cannot be considered *simply* medical treatment. Christian theology provides a moral context for the discussion. Eating is a moral responsibility for image bearers of God. The beating of our hearts and the functioning of our kidneys are not moral tasks, but God regulated human eating at creation as part of man's basic responsibility to have dominion over the earth and to work and to guard the garden (Gen. 1:26–29; 2:9, 15–17). He also cursed (and sustained) fallen humanity in their eating (Gen. 3:17–19), and he again regulated human eating after the flood (Gen. 9:2–4). In addition to all of this, many sacramental rituals in both Old and New Testaments involved eating, and the life of the heavenly kingdom is described as a banquet (Matt. 22:2; Rev. 19:9). Hence we must be careful never to equate the requirement of food and drink to satisfy hunger and thirst with, for example, the need for dialysis to compensate for failing kidneys or for insulin to compensate for a deficient pancreas. Yet this biblical material also reminds us that eating is inseparable from the larger task of exercising dominion over this world as God's image bearers, and the complete and permanent inability of the PVS patient to grow, prepare, chew, and swallow his food highlights how much this person lacks ordinary human characteristics. This observation is not meant to challenge the affirmation of his human personhood, but it does strengthen the case that providing ANH for PVS patients cannot be considered *merely* ordinary care for a feeble individual. ANH should not be simplistically deemed basic care only or medical treatment only.

I suggest that we need not be detained by the "care versus treatment" debate when trying to make a morally responsible decision about ANH. Even though there may be a higher burden for forgoing nutrition and hydration than for forgoing chemotherapy or even dialysis, for reasons just considered, the guidelines offered earlier in this chapter suggest that there are times even when food and drink may be refused. We ought not to forgo food and drink for the purpose of bringing death, which is a form of suicide. But the absence of suffering and physical hardship is a valuable human good. Though we are called to endure suffering, we are not obligated to torment ourselves. When food and drink are revolting, they may be refused. A person may choose to forgo eating in order to enjoy a better (though shorter) life than the kind of life that he would have to endure if he continued to eat.

It is worth investigating whether these considerations help us in the case of a PVS patient, for there is perhaps no other way to get to the bottom of this question. A good place to begin this investigation is by reflecting on the answer of Gilbert Meilaender, who makes the most convincing and winsome case of which I am aware against forgoing ANH for the PVS patient. Meilaender argues that providing ANH to this patient cannot be considered burdensome to him. The PVS patient does not experience pain or discomfort of any sort, and thus the insertion and maintenance of a feeding tube inflicts no suffering. His life itself may be burdensome, Meilaender argues, but we are never to choose to end life because it is hard. Since the provision of ANH itself is not a burden but benefits the life that the patient has, then ANH should be provided because it is a choice of life over death.

Key to Meilaender's argument is the claim that providing ANH itself is not a burden to the unconscious patient. It is difficult to argue with this claim. But the very thing that makes this claim persuasive makes the second key component of his argument questionable. If the PVS patient is not burdened by the treatment because of his inability to experience anything, then is it persuasive to conclude that the treatment "benefits the life the patient has"? How exactly does the provision of ANH benefit the life of such a patient, who experiences nothing at all? The ANH obviously *sustains* the life, but that is not the same thing as benefiting "the life that he has." To insist that the mere sustaining of life is a benefit seems to beg the question. One of the chief claims of this chapter—with which Meilaender himself agrees—is that the mere sustaining of life is not the highest human good, which is the very reason why people may justly decide to forgo treatment in certain situations. A permanently unconscious patient, for as long as he lives, experiences neither benefit nor burden from ANH.

Some readers may be persuaded by Meilaender, and if so then their conclusion must be that ANH should always be provided for PVS patients. But if Meilaender's argument falls just short, then how can we resolve this question? I suggest that we should again attempt to evaluate this question in terms of a choice between two kinds of life, rather than as a choice between life and death. Looking at this question merely in terms of earthly goods puts us at a moral standstill. Whether this person lives a shorter life without ANH or a longer life with ANH, his permanently unconscious state makes neither life the better life. Either way there is no pain or pleasure, sorrow or joy, accomplishment or failure. Another way to find resolution may be to turn to the larger social dynamics at work in the particular situation and to assess the benefits and burdens of continuing the treatment upon family and friends. Continuing ANH may be a great financial burden on families in some cases, but may also provide a meaningful occasion for loved ones to express compassion, care, and self-sacrifice in helping the weak. Again there is nothing morally decisive that resolves the question.

But what if we look at this question, finally, with respect to spiritual goods? Taking this perspective will make sense only in the case of Christians caring for Christians. Christians are united to Christ and called to embrace him in faith and to honor him with prayer and worship. Yet the PVS patient is unable to engage in these activities to which he is called. Though ANH is neither burdensome nor beneficial with respect to earthly goods, it seems reasonable to characterize it as spiritually burdensome, for its very purpose is to keep someone in a state of existence in which he is unable to fulfill his religious responsibilities and privileges. To put the question again: which life is a better life for the Christian, the shorter life without ANH or the longer life with ANH? To conclude that the shorter life is the better life is a morally sound choice, in my judgment, because it recognizes that this shorter life does not have to endure treatment that serves to prohibit conscious communion with Christ. I hasten to add, however, that this is not a choice that I would force upon another person's conscience.

Conclusion

Death is our enemy and no one should wish to face it for its own sake. Yet the advent of modern medical technology compels us to consider when it is time to cease fighting death and to forgo further treatment. Sometimes these ethical questions have easy answers, but often they do not. Death comes for us all, and its approach cannot be kept at bay forever, however remarkable medical technology has become. Because Christians know that earthly life is not the highest good and that death is a defeated enemy, they may make decisions to forgo treatment without a sense of despair and defeat, however difficult these decisions often are because of the complexity of the situation and the lack of explicit biblical teaching. Christians do not choose death, but they may choose a shorter life with the confidence that one day the Lord Jesus Christ "will transform our lowly body to be like his glorious body, by the power that enables him even to subject all things to himself" (Phil. 3:21).

CONCLUSION
(WITH A BIBLIOGRAPHIC ESSAY)

At the beginning of this book I observed that moral issues about life and death are perennial. Carrying a child in the womb, dealing with an illness, and facing the prospect of death can be defining events in a person's life. They challenge us to act nobly and tempt us to act basely. In a fallen world these experiences are constitutive for human existence and put our theory and practice of ethics to the test.

These things are as true for early twenty-first-century Christians as they have been for others throughout history, but twenty-first-century Christians face such issues in two distinctive ways. First, with their nonbelieving contemporaries, they now confront matters of life and death and health and illness with access to medical technology unimaginable even in the recent past. With this technology diseases can be fought and life preserved in ways enormously beneficial to the human race. Yet these technological advancements have not changed the basic ethical questions surrounding life and death, but have in fact compounded and complicated these questions by giving human beings newly realized powers and possibilities. Second, twenty-first-century Christians, with their fellow believers of all generations, confront matters of life and death and health and illness not simply as fallen sinners living in a cursed but preserved world. Because of the life, death, and resurrection of the Lord Jesus Christ, the curse of death has been lifted and they have the hope of everlasting life in the age to come. They now live, suffer, and die in ways that are radically different from the ways of the world. Their new life in Christ does not make bioethical questions easy, but it does bring a transformed perspective and blessed encouragement in the face of what can be the darkest and weightiest moments of human life.

This book, written for Christians in an early twenty-first-century context, has sought to take account of these various dimensions of bioethics: the perennial challenges of life, illness, and death as rooted in our common human nature, the new challenges sparked by the explosion of contemporary medical technology, and the transformed perspective on these matters that comes through faith in Christ. Though there are many significant bioethical issues that I have not had opportunity to address, I have sought to set forth a way of Christian thinking and living that prepares believers to navigate through the modern world's bioethics maze. It is my hope that readers will grow in their understanding and practice of the doctrines and virtues discussed in these pages and thereby handle their own bioethical challenges in ways that are increasingly wise, responsible, neighbor-benefiting, and God-glorifying. I also hope that some readers who share the basic convictions animating this volume will research and reflect upon some of the many bioethical questions that I have not specifically addressed and be able to provide additional insight for believers who are grappling with these matters.

For those who wish to do more reading on particular issues, I conclude this book with the following bibliographic essay. This essay will provide information about the articles and books that I have referred to in this volume and also mention some other literature that is important or helpful. It is certainly not comprehensive, but should provide many leads for curious readers who want to dig more deeply into the fascinating world of bioethics.

A Bibliographic Essay

Two books are worth mentioning at the outset, Gilbert Meilaender's *Bioethics: A Primer for Christians* (Grand Rapids, MI: Eerdmans, 1996) and Leon R. Kass's *Life, Liberty and the Defense of Dignity* (San Francisco: Encounter, 2002). Both books cover a broad range of bioethical issues and could have been mentioned at various points below as providing grist for further reading. Meilaender is a Lutheran ethicist. I have found his book to be a very helpful brief introduction to bioethics from a theological perspective similar though not identical to my own. Kass is a medical doctor who has served as a professor at the University of Chicago and as the chairman of the President's Council on Bioethics. I have found Kass's work to be stimulating and challenging in all sorts of ways, though he does not write from a theological perspective. I have learned much about bioethics from these two books and from other things that these authors have written, and I recommend them to others.

In chapter 1 I described a number of different approaches to the question of how Christian conviction ought to shape the bioethics enterprise. Readers should remember that the five categories that I used to describe these different approaches are categories of my own invention, designed as a pedagogical aid, and not the self-described categories of any of the authors that I mentioned. Among important works that I place in the *secular bioethics only* category are Tom L. Beauchamp and James F. Childress, *Principles of Biomedical Ethics*, 5th ed. (New York: Oxford University Press, 2001); Robert M. Veatch, *A Theory of Medical Ethics* (New York: Basic Books, 1981); and Robert M. Veatch, *The Basics of Bioethics*, 2nd ed. (Upper Saddle River, NJ: Prentice Hall, 2003). These three writers have been very influential in the broader world of bioethics over the last several decades. I mentioned two authors in connection with the *Christian bioethics only* category, John Frame and Marsha Fowler. The works on which I based my comments about them are John M. Frame, *Medical Ethics: Principles, Persons, and Problems* (Phillipsburg, NJ: Presbyterian and Reformed, 1988) and Marsha D. Fowler, "Christian Teaching and the Church's Authority," in *Bioengagement: Making a Christian Difference through Bioethics Today*, ed. Nigel M. de S. Cameron, Scott E. Daniels, and Barbara J. White (Grand Rapids, MI: Eerdmans, 2000), 235–48.

I associated the *secular and Christian bioethics identical* category with a number of Roman Catholic ethicists. Those that I mentioned are among the most influential bioethics scholars in Roman Catholic circles in recent years. Their works which I quoted in chapter 1 are Richard A. McCormick, "Bioethics and method: Where do we start?" *Theology Digest* 29 (Winter 1981): 303–18; Lisa Sowle Cahill, *Theological Bioethics: Participation, Justice, and Change* (Washington, DC: Georgetown University Press, 2005); and James J. Walter and Thomas A. Shannon, *Contemporary Issues in Bioethics: A Catholic Perspective* (Lanham: Rowman & Littlefield, 2005). The two major works in which H. Tristram Engelhardt Jr. sets forth his approach to bioethics, which I labeled *secular and Christian bioethics radically different*, are

The Foundations of Bioethics, 2nd ed. (New York: Oxford University Press, 1996) and *The Foundations of Christian Bioethics* (Lisse: Swets & Zeitlinger, 2000). I mentioned a number of writers as representing various formulations of the approach entitled *secular bioethics and Christian bioethics distinct but legitimate.* Two Roman Catholic scholars, Edmund D. Pellegrino and David C. Thomasma, are coauthors of two volumes that I noted, *The Virtues in Medical Practice* (New York: Oxford University Press, 1993) and *The Christian Virtues in Medical Practice* (Washington, DC: Georgetown University Press, 1996). Among Protestant writers the following works are relevant: John Jefferson Davis, *Evangelical Ethics*, 3rd ed. (Phillipsburg, NJ: P&R, 2004) and Scott B. Rae and Paul M. Cox, *Bioethics: A Christian Approach in a Pluralistic Age* (Grand Rapids, MI: Eerdmans, 1999). Another distinctive approach that also belongs somewhere in this category is found in Joel Shuman and Brian Volck, *Reclaiming the Body: Christians and the Faithful Use of Modern Medicine* (Grand Rapids, MI: Brazos, 2006).

Some readers may be interested in the development of the discipline of bioethics, which is relatively new as a distinct academic pursuit. Two works that deal with this are Albert R. Jonsen, *The Birth of Bioethics* (New York: Oxford University Press, 2003) and *The Story of Bioethics: From Seminal Works to Contemporary Explorations*, ed. Jennifer K. Walter and Eran P. Klein (Washington, DC: Georgetown University Press, 2003).

My own approach to the relationship of secular and Christian bioethics and to the more general question of the Christian's relationship to the mainstream health-care system reflects both the "two cities" theology of Augustine of Hippo (set forth in his magisterial *The City of God*) and the "two kingdoms" theology of the Reformation, especially in its Reformed expression. For more on the historical roots of my approach, see David VanDrunen, *Natural Law and the Two Kingdoms: A Study in the Development of Reformed Social Thought* (Grand Rapids, MI: Eerdmans, forthcoming). I have developed some of the broader biblical and theological principles underlying my argument in chapter 3 of *A Biblical Case for Natural Law* (Grand Rapids, MI: Acton Institute, 2006).

Chapter 2 discusses a number of important Christian doctrines that have special relevance for bioethics. For those wishing to explore Christian doctrine more generally I recommend John Calvin's *Institutes of the Christian Religion*, 2 vols., ed. J. T. McNeill, trans. F. L. Battles

(Philadelphia: Westminster, 1960) as a classic and unparalleled exposition. Among subsequent works that remain very helpful, in ascending order of size and thoroughness, are Louis Berkhof, *Manual of Christian Doctrine* (Grand Rapids, MI: Eerdmans, 1998); Louis Berkhof, *Systematic Theology: New Combined Edition* (Grand Rapids, MI: Eerdmans, 1996); and Herman Bavinck, *Reformed Dogmatics*, 4 vols., ed. John Bolt, trans. John Vriend (Grand Rapids, MI: Baker, 2003–2008).

The question of suffering is an especially difficult one, and in that light I am happy to commend two recent books by colleagues at Westminster Seminary California which consider issues of suffering in a theologically sound and pastorally sensitive manner: Michael Horton, *Too Good to Be True: Finding Hope in a World of Hype* (Grand Rapids, MI: Zondervan, 2006) and Hywel R. Jones, *A Study Commentary on Job* (Darlington, England: Evangelical Press, 2007). From a very different perspective, a recent book explores the vanity of American obsession with earthly happiness and the meaningfulness of suffering for ordinary human experience: Eric G. Wilson, *Against Happiness: In Praise of Melancholy* (New York: Farrar, Straus and Giroux, 2008).

At the end of chapter 2 I mentioned transhumanism, which looks to genetic engineering to create a post-human species with enhanced capabilities and lifespan. Among books promoting various forms of transhumanism are Ronald Bailey, *Liberation Biology: The Scientific and Moral Case for the Biotech Revolution* (New York: Prometheus, 2005) and Ray Kurzweil, *The Singularity Is Near: When Humans Transcend Biology* (New York: Penguin, 2006). Books by prominent authors that are critical of transhumanism include Francis Fukuyama, *Our Posthuman Future: Consequences of the Biotechnology Revolution* (New York: Picador, 2002) and the President's Council on Bioethics (chaired by Leon R. Kass), *Beyond Therapy: Biotechnology and the Pursuit of Happiness* (Washington, DC: The President's Council on Bioethics, 2003).

I considered various Christian virtues in chapter 3. I mentioned that through most of Western history philosophers and theologians writing about ethics ordinarily viewed virtues as a very important part of the discussion. Classic philosophical works from pre-Christian times that presented influential accounts of the virtues are Plato's *Republic* and Aristotle's *Nicomachean Ethics* (both available in various editions). Perhaps the Christian theologian best known for his exposition of the virtues is Thomas Aquinas, particularly in the Second Part of his *Summa Theologiae* (also available in various editions), though many other Protestant and Roman Catholic theologians also pursued the subject of virtue. For one example of a Puritan exploration of a virtue discussed in chapter 3, see Jeremiah Burroughs, *The Rare Jewel of Christian Contentment* (Edinburgh: Banner of Truth, 1992). The modern renaissance of thinking about virtue was primarily initiated by Alistair MacIntyre's *After Virtue: A Study in Moral Theory* (Notre Dame: University of Notre Dame Press, 1981). Two notable Protestants who have done significant thinking about virtue ethics are Stanley Hauerwas and Gilbert Meilaender. Among their relevant works, see Stanley Hauerwas, *Vision and Virtue: Essays in Christian Ethical Reflection* (Notre Dame: University of Notre Dame Press, 1981) and Gilbert Meilaender, *The Theory and Practice of Virtue* (Notre Dame: University of Notre Dame Press, 1988).

Chapter 3 concluded with a discussion of wisdom. Two helpful studies on the biblical wisdom literature are William P. Brown, *Character in Crisis: A Fresh Approach to the Wisdom Literature of the Old Testament* (Grand Rapids, MI: Eerdmans, 1996) and Roland E. Murphy, *The Tree of Life: An Exploration of Biblical Wisdom Literature*, 3rd ed. (Grand Rapids, MI: Eerdmans, 2002).

Part 2 dealt with beginning of life bioethics issues. A number of books by evangelical authors consider the issues investigated in these chapters (4–6), including J. P. Moreland and Scott B. Rae, *Body & Soul: Human Nature & the Crisis in Ethics* (Downers Grove: InterVarsity, 2000) and Edwin C. Hui, *At the Beginning of Life: Dilemmas in Theological Bioethics* (Downers Grove: InterVarsity, 2002). From a somewhat different theological perspective is the concise, but challenging and insightful, treatment of these beginning-of-life issues by the Anglican moral theologian Oliver O'Donovan in *Begotten or Made?* (Oxford: Clarendon, 1984). For official Roman Catholic teaching on various beginning-of-life issues, see *Humanae Vitae*, the 1987 Instruction issued by the Congregation for the Doctrine of the Faith, which is easily accessible on the Vatican's Web site. For an example of a book written by Protestants critical of artificial contraception, see Sam & Bethany Torode, *Open Embrace: A Protestant Couple Rethinks Contraception* (Grand Rapids, MI: Eerdmans, 2002). This book advocates use of natural family planning and contains further information about it. For opposing arguments about whether the Pill causes abortions, written by authors who share pro-life sentiments, see *The Reproductive Revolution: A Christian Appraisal of Sexuality, Reproductive Technologies, and the Family*, ed. John F. Kliner, Paige C. Cunningham, and W. David Hager (Grand Rapids, MI: Eerdmans, 2000), chapter 10.

A great deal of material has been written, of course, on the status of the human embryo and at what point the embryo becomes a human person. In addition to many books cited above which defend a position similar to the one that I defend in chapter 6, I mention a recent, rigorously argued contribution to the literature: Robert P. George and Christopher Tollefsen, *Embryo: A Defense of Human Life* (New York: Doubleday, 2008). An article that I cite favorably in chapter 6 is Meredith G. Kline, "*Lex Talionis* and the Human Fetus," *Journal of the Evangelical Theological Society* 20 (September 1977): 193–201. A number of books and articles have made theological arguments against the view that human personhood begins at fertilization. For an example of a Roman Catholic argument that individuality and hence personhood does not begin until about three weeks after fertilization, see the essay by Thomas Shannon and Allan B. Wolter, "Reflections on the Moral Status of the Pre-embryo" in *Contemporary Issues in Bioethics*, edited by Walter and Shannon, cited above. For an example of a mainline Protestant argument advocating embryonic stem-cell research, see Ted Peters, *The Stem Cell Debate* (Minneapolis: Fortress, 2007).

Part 3 considered matters pertaining to death and dying. In chapter 7 I mentioned a number of books written over the past sixty years that reflect the shift in thinking about death in mainstream American culture: John Gunther, *Death Be Not Proud: A Memoir* (1949; New York: HarperPerennial, 1989); Elisabeth Kübler-Ross, *On Death and Dying* (New York: Macmillan, 1969); Sherwin Nuland, *How We Die: Reflections on Life's Final Chapter* (New York: Knopf, 1994); and Ira Byock, *Dying Well: Peace and Possibilities at the End of Life* (New York: Riverhead, 1997). I also mentioned the best-seller by Randy Pausch (with Jeffrey Zaslow) written after his diagnosis with terminal pancreatic cancer, *The Last Lecture* (New York: Hyperion, 2008). A few works that deal with the *ars moriendi* tradition are David William Atkinson, *The English Ars Moriendi* (New York: Peter Lang, 1992); Christopher P. Voigt, *Patience, Compassion, Hope, and the Christian Art of Dying Well* (Lanham, MD: Rowman & Littlefield, 2004); and Austra Reinis, *Reforming the Art of Dying: The Ars Moriendi in the German Reformation (1519–1528)* (Aldershot, England: Ashgate, 2007).

Many theological works have reflected upon death, and I mention only a few of them, from various theological perspectives. Among books by Protestant writers are Helmut Thielicke, *Death and Life*, trans. Edward H. Schroeder (Philadelphia: Fortress, 1970) and Eberhard Jüngel, *Death: The Riddle and the Mystery*, trans. Iain and Ute Nicol (Philadelphia: Westminster, 1974). Significant Roman Catholic works include Josef Pieper, *Death and Immortality*, trans. Richard and Clara Winston (New York: Herder and Herder, 1969); Karl Rahner, *On the Theology of Death* (New York: Seabury, 1973); and Richard John Neuhaus, *As I Lay Dying: Meditations upon Returning* (New York: Basic, 2002). An Eastern Orthodox perspective on death is presented in Vigen Guroian, *Life's Living toward Dying: A Theological and Medical-Ethical Study* (Grand Rapids, MI: Eerdmans, 1996). Readers of novels know that many novels explore issues of death and dying very profoundly. Perhaps most noteworthy is Leo Tolstoy's *The Death of Ivan Ilyich*, trans. Lynn Solotaroff (New York: Bantam, 1981).

A great amount of literature also exists on euthanasia and physician-assisted suicide, issues discussed in chapter 8. One recent study that puts these matters in helpful historical perspective is Ian Dowbiggin, *A Concise History of Euthanasia: Life, Death, God, and Medicine* (Lanham, MD: Rowman & Littlefield, 2005). A number of essays from a Christian perspective in critique of euthanasia appear in *Death without Dignity: Euthanasia in Perspective*, ed. Nigel M. de S. Cameron (Edinburgh: Rutherford House, 1990). Essays that also critique euthanasia, but written from a nonreligious secular perspective, are found in *The Case against Assisted Suicide: For the Right to End-of-Life Care*, ed. Kathleen Foley, M.D., and Herbert Hendin, M.D. (Baltimore: Johns Hopkins University Press, 2002). In chapter 8 I also interacted with an influential argument by James Rachels rejecting the idea that there is a significant moral distinction between *killing* and *letting die*. His argument appears in "Euthanasia, Killing, and Letting Die," in *Medical Responsibility: Paternalism, Informed Consent, and Euthanasia* (Clifton, NJ: Humana, 1979), 153–68.

One of the effective voices responding to arguments like Rachels's is that of Daniel Callahan, whom I interact with in chapters 8 and 9. Though his book *The Troubled Dream of Life: Living with Mortality* (New York: Simon & Schuster, 1993) is not written from a Christian perspective it is well worth reading. The article by Gilbert Meilaender, "Living Life's End," in the May 2005 *First Things*, was influential in developing my own views about the difference between choosing death and choosing different kinds of life, as reflected in chapters

8 and 9. This article also sets forth Meilaender's argument against withdrawing artificial nutrition and hydration from PVS patients. For competing Roman Catholic views on the PVS question, see the essays in *Artificial Nutrition and Hydration and the Permanently Unconscious Patient: The Catholic Debate*, ed. Ronald P. Hamel and James J. Walter (Washington, DC: Georgetown University Press, 2007).

General Index

Scripture Index